SAVING STELLA

SAVING STELLA

•

Notes from a Nurse Turned Legislator

SHIRLEY NATHAN-PULLIAM

JOHNS HOPKINS UNIVERSITY PRESS | *Baltimore*

© 2024 Johns Hopkins University Press
All rights reserved. Published 2024
Printed in the United States of America on acid-free paper
9 8 7 6 5 4 3 2 1

Johns Hopkins University Press
2715 North Charles Street
Baltimore, Maryland 21218
www.press.jhu.edu

Library of Congress Cataloging-in-Publication Data

Names: Nathan-Pulliam, Shirley, 1939– author.
Title: Saving Stella : notes from a nurse turned legislator / by Shirley
    Nathan-Pulliam.
Description: Baltimore : Johns Hopkins University Press, 2024. | Includes
    bibliographical references and index.
Identifiers: LCCN 2023033242 | ISBN 9781421448862 (hardcover ; alk. paper) |
    ISBN 9781421448879 (ebook)
Subjects: MESH: Nathan-Pulliam, Shirley, 1939– | Nurses | Healthcare Disparities—
    legislation & jurisprudence | Political Activism | Social Determinants of Health |
    Health Policy | Emigrants and Immigrants | Maryland | United States |
    Autobiography
Classification: LCC RT37.N37 | NLM WZ 100 | DDC 610.73092—dc23/eng/20231106
LC record available at https://lccn.loc.gov/2023033242

A catalog record for this book is available from the British Library.

*Special discounts are available for bulk purchases of this book. For more information,
please contact Special Sales at specialsales@jh.edu.*

To my children Wayne, Sharon, and Warren

*My grandchildren Brianna, Nicole, Warren Jr.,
Jaye-Ann, and Maya*

*And most specifically to my great-granddaughter,
Zoey Lee Faulkner*

Brothers Lloyd and Nicholas

Sisters Valerie and Harlene

Of all the forms of inequality, injustice in health care is
the most shocking and the most inhumane.
—DR. MARTIN LUTHER KING JR., 1965

CONTENTS

This book is the fascinating and compelling life story of a strong Jamaican woman who displays indomitable courage, perseverance, strength of character, and remarkable compassion with the plight of others in the many roles she has played. The story unfolds in three parts, which are separated in time but are clearly linked together and influence each other.

The first act is played out in Jamaica. Those older persons who have lived in Jamaica or those who have read or listened to stories of the good old days will become misty-eyed at the pictures that are painted. Those were the days when a little girl named Shirley Nathan could travel unafraid from Montego Bay to Kingston by train—when the dead were buried in caskets made from their own mahogany trees and large families were the norm, with children having "Aunties" in multiple households. But underpinning this apparently idyllic life was the fact that little Shirley was dyslexic, ridiculed by her father for being backward, failing in formal schooling, and apparently destined for a life of non-achievement by conventional standards. We get a glimpse even then of a characteristic that would mark her life. She had a firm and abiding faith in her own capability and lived a maxim that she would verbalize as an adult: "Can't is not in my vocabulary." She tells the story of working to obtain the money for her passage to England to study nursing to the surprise of a doubting Papa.

The second act is a relatively short period spent in England, where she completed her nursing education, overcoming or rather coping with dyslexia by dint of concentration and application. She met and fell in love with an American soldier. They were married when she was twenty-one years old.

Then begins the concluding act as she comes to America. There are graphic descriptions of the culture shock—differences in accommodation; the experiences of racial segregation and discrimination; struggles to make a living and having to train as a practical nurse, teaching others less qualified than she was. Shirley is gloriously gregarious by nature and finds an outlet for her energy in becoming a community activist, joining numerous organizations, boards, and commissions, while also going to school and taking care of a family—with a marriage that was dissolving.

It is here that we begin to see the kindling, or perhaps fanning, of the fire that characterizes this latter part of her life. Shirley comes to grips with the impact of social conditions on health and begins to appreciate the real meaning of the quote she cites from Martin Luther King Jr.: "Of all the forms of inequality, injustice in health care is the most shocking and the most inhumane because it often results in physical death." There is a palpable feeling of injustice in the fact that Stella died in the late stages of breast cancer because her social condition denied her that early diagnosis and treatment that would have been the norm for those endowed with the necessary material resources.

It is the crusade—and that is the appropriate word—for equity in health outcomes that is the driving passion of Shirley's later years. She realizes that the personal care of nursing is indispensable at the individual level, but if she is to help and save the many, then the phrase of Rudolf Virchow, the German physician / political activist, is apt. Virchow famously said: "Medicine is a social science and politics is nothing else but medicine on a grand scale." Shirley tells of entry into elective politics, the alliances she had to form, her initial defeat at the polls, and her subsequent success in 1994 when she was elected to the Maryland General Assembly, the first Jamaican or Caribbean person to be elected to that body in its over 300 years of existence. One cannot fail to be enthralled by the description of the awe that struck her when she realized what she had accomplished, and how she was moved by the history and tradition of which she was now a part. She brought to her task the habits cultivated over a lifetime, and undoubtedly her nursing training was a good background—problem identification, development of the plan, implementation, follow-up, and evaluation. Her learning curve was steep and sometimes rocky. She had to put in an enormous amount of work to keep up with the rapidly evolving legislative issues. She served in the Maryland House of Delegates for twenty years until she was elected to the state senate in 2014 for the first of two terms.

There are gripping accounts of the political battles she fought, the bills she introduced, and the alliances needed to get her legislation passed. The politics of government is said to be an art, and she became a wizard at it. Appreciation that legislators are more prone to collaborate when they are personally affected and her conclusion that there was little interest among legislators in really understanding the root causes of health disparities give some insight into the tactics she had to use to accomplish her legislative victories.

The emphasis on health and health care shines throughout the book, but there is clear recognition that to address the disparities one must look at the social determinants of health. In addition, it is salutary to see the appreciation that health care is not synonymous with health. Health is important not only in its own right as one of the capabilities that contribute to and enhance the quality of life, but health is also instrumental. It is essential for education, as she appreciates in sponsoring legislation on education, but in addition, a healthy life has economic dimensions, and the long life that accompanies health allows for increased returns on investment in education. Health disparities are important as they show the differences between groups, but as Shirley points out, inequity represents the unfair and avoidable differences that are beyond the agency of the disadvantaged. Many factors serve as discriminators of inequity, and this book deals with several, including race, poverty, and social situation.

No autobiography is complete without a window into the persona of the author, and Shirley does not hide the many trials and travails of her life. She is open about her personal illness and about her son's dyslexia and addiction, but rather than moping about these, she uses them as the impetus to direct some of her legislative fire toward public measures for their alleviation. She is also open about her personal achievements, her academic qualifications—bachelor's and master's degrees—and her business acumen in starting and running successful health care enterprises. The book is also replete with the names of the many friends who helped her at various and often difficult times.

She has been lauded and applauded in numerous fora of distinction. Awards are numerous, and her legislative battles as champion of eliminating social injustice with its negative impact on the poor and dispossessed have been appropriately recognized by her peers. It was fitting that her legislative work was honored by a bill in the Maryland State Assembly entitled The Shirley Nathan-Pulliam Health Equity Act of 2021. But in reading this book, one notes that its pages are haunted by the fact that Stella was not saved. A counterpoint is the passion and compassion Shirley Nathan Pulliam exhibits in trying to ensure that there are fewer or perhaps no Stellas in the years to come.

The book is well written and researched, with some of the health issues explained in a manner that would give credit to a good school of public health. This is a fascinating read, and I recommend it unreservedly to all those who wish for a better world and look for an example of one who tries to make it so. And as she writes pithily at the end, "I am not finished yet."

—SIR GEORGE ALLEYNE
Chancellor and Emeritus Professor, University of the West Indies
Director Emeritus, Pan American Health Organization

ACKNOWLEDGMENTS

Many people have touched my life through various stages and helped shape me into the person I have become. My deepest thanks to all who have given me guidance and sustained me in myriad ways.

My particular thanks to Rector Florence Ledyard of St. Bartholomew's Episcopal Church and Cannon Kortright Davis, a retired Episcopal priest, and to my friend of almost sixty years, Inez Haynie Dobson—all of whom I admire and who continue to give me spiritual guidance.

This book would not have been written without the help and encouragement of many. Special thanks to Donna Hemans, who helped with the preparation of the manuscript; Sir George Alleyne, MD, former chancellor of the University of the West Indies, for writing the foreword; literary agent Sha-Shana Crichton, Esq.; Margaret Bernal and Queen Ayacodobae, who for years encouraged me to write my memoirs; the late Harriet Bais Branch, who was my friend and study partner; and Dr. Louise Johnson and Dr. Elaine Simon, for our work in the Black Women Consciousness Raising Association (BWCRA).

Thanks to my colleagues in the Maryland General Assembly who affected my life during my tenure. A special thanks to President of the Senate Bill Ferguson, Speaker of the House Adrienne Jones, and Senator Delores Kelley, whose ticket I was privileged to join early in my political career. I am particularly grateful to former Speaker of the House Mike Bush and former President of the Senate Mike Miller (both deceased), and Delegate Peter Hammen, former chair, Health and Government Operations Committee, who all gave me a chance to grow. I would also like to recognize the other legislators who were also originally from the Caribbean: State Senator Arthur Ellis (Jamaica), Delegates Gabriel Acevero (Trinidad and Tobago), Regina Boyce (Barbados and Jamaica), Joseline Peña-Melnyk, chair, Health and Government Operations Committee (Dominican Republic), and Jheanelle Wilkins (Jamaica).

I am enormously grateful to my campaign manager, Kenny Brown, who has been my friend and a brother through our many years of successful campaigning; my first campaign treasurer, the late Dr. Dorothy E. Brunson; my brother, Nicholas Baron Nathan, who also served as treasurer of my campaign; Albert Annan, the longest-serving and immediate past treasurer, and Dr. Lennox Graham, chair, of Friends of Shirley Nathan-Pulliam; and the delegate representing the Virgin Islands in Congress, Donna Christensen, MD, for our work on health disparities with the Congressional Black Caucus (CBC) Health Brain Trust (HBT).

A special thanks to Millicent McLeod, my best girlfriend and confidante of over fifty years, who was always there for me—whether fixing a meal, calling to ensure I was okay, reminding me of the fabulous times and educational experiences we've had, or attending conferences and parties throughout the years. My thanks to Dalverine West-Aarons, RN, nurse practitioner, whom I met as a constituent and who became my friend and nurse and looked out for me on a daily basis. Antoinette Mugar, RN, MS, who took care of my health whenever I needed her. My three nursing girlfriends who stuck with me while I was trying to start my adult medical day care—Gwendolyn Jacobs, Sarah Williams, and Milda Lewis—and Henry Burris, retired firefighter. My gratitude to my friend Avril Johnson, who showed up time after time at my hotel in Annapolis with some good Jamaican food and company to soothe my spirit. A big thank-you to Andrene Bonner (author and friend); Carmen Nelson Edwards for her wisdom; Rick Nugent, my partner in creating the Jamaican Association of Maryland; Alice Torriente, for keeping me informed on political issues daily; and Pauline Watson, a longtime friend and supporter. Alease Cobb and Nicole Earle, who have both been so generous to me and looked out for me.

I am also grateful to Dr. Carlessia Hussein, with whom I bonded over our shared concerns about public health issues that impact racial and ethnic disparities, as well as our concerns and thoughts as parents for our children and grandchildren; and Fredette West, for her fighting spirit and ongoing efforts to make life better for our people.

A big thank-you to Albert Reece, MD, former dean of the University of Maryland School of Medicine, and his wife, Sharon Reece, associate professor at the University of Maryland School of Law, for their friendship and for being a go-to whenever there was a health crisis involving my constituents or myself or when I needed advice. I am grateful to Dr. Jane Kirschling, dean of the University of Maryland School of Nursing, for believing in and promoting me and my work. A special thanks to Jay A. Perman, MD, chancellor of the University System of Maryland, for caring about my community.

My deepest gratitude to former Baltimore City Community College professor Dr. Doris Starks (later the dean of Coppin State University School of Nursing), who has always recognized me as one who added feathers in her hat every time I accomplished something new, as well as professors Francis Hicks-Gordon and Gertrude Hodgers, who gave me an opportunity to start the nursing program even though I was one month late. My sincerest gratitude to my consultant and friend, Dr. Mary Etta Mills, who taught me about writing standards of care and encouraged me to go back to college for a higher degree.

There is a special place in my heart for my "adopted" children. The order in which their names appear does not represent their place in my heart. Wanda Belle, who was my researcher through my political campaign and a former legislative assistant; Roger Clark, whom I called my son and who looked out for and chauffeured and supported me through the years of political campaigning to the present time; Larry Gourdine, Eric Tharrington, Terri Wilson (goddaughter), Marie Anthony, Dino Rodwell, Troy Riveria, Joan Dunning, Regina Clark, Donni Glover, Bishop Barry Chapman, and Haki Ammi; Dr. Tyrone and Jean Taborn, for exposing me to the outstanding accomplishments of our people through the Black Engineers of the Year Award; Dr. Goulda

Downer, for her excellent way of accomplishing whatever task was at hand and her role in the Caribbean Political Action Pact; Dr. Claire Nelson, founder of the Institute of Caribbean Studies; Fandreia Bowman, Donavan Murphy, and Camile Quinlan, who made sure I was not hungry when I was recuperating from surgery; Tracee Bryant Hall, Annelle Primm, MD, and Joseph Daniels, who helped me with my mental health during trying times; Dr. Yolanda Ogbolu, a feather in my hat; Dr. Maurice Miles, Dr. Trudy Hall, Dr. Charlotte Wood, and Dr. Hyacinth Dunstant-Hunte, who have always made me so very proud; Kim Anderson Mack, who checks on me almost daily; Dr. William "Bill" Johnson, who cared tremendously about my health; and my adopted grandchildren—Kameron Nelson, Ty Taborn (both exceptional legislative interns), Zoey Aarons, Tendai Murray, and Hanna Murray.

My campaign staff, managers, and legislative aides each have a special place in my heart: campaign manager and legislative aide Adetoun Olumide, Esq.; legislative aides Sue Ann Sontesifer, Lydia Sampson, Pam Hall, and Thomas Cover; and chiefs of staff Eli Berns Zeve, Esq., Joshua Hoffman, Esq., Evan Johnson, and Elaine Zammett. My gratitude to Delegate Jim Campbell and Delegate Sandy Rosenberg, for allowing me to run my first race on their ticket; and to Catherine E. Pugh, former mayor of Baltimore who worked on my first campaign and served with me on the Hub Board and in the state senate of Maryland.

My gratitude to Charlee Mclean, MD, whose sheer drive and tenacity are unmatched; Christopher Gibbons, MD, for genuinely caring about others; Basil Morgan, MD, and Athol Morgan, MD, for always being there for me whatever the situation brings; Majid Hussain and Jai and Dr. Hollis Sinerine, businessmen, friends, and longtime contributors to the Friends of Shirley Nathan-Pulliam; Sharon Solomon, MD, Johns Hopkins University, for her clinical excellence; Myron L. Weisfeldt, MD, Improving Health Outcomes and Medical Education and Sickle Cell Disease Network; Sophie Lanzkron, MD, researcher at John Hopkins University; and Dr. Franklin Knight, professor emeritus, historian, of Johns Hopkins University.

My gratitude to Larry Weston, author and my first-grade friend from Mico Practicing School in Kingston, Jamaica, whom I still call on for ideas regularly; and Ambassador Curtis Ward, my friend and mentor.

Thanks to my Florida friends, old and new: Patrecia Hines (who has given her time and love to caring for people), Shirley Edwards, RN, BSN, Carmen Gewirtz, Gussie Lovelle Fequiere, RN, Ronie and Steven Pall, James and Pilar Schuitema, Anita Marcelle, Yvonne Tai-sen Choy, Carl and Elease Ruddock, Aldena Clifford, Rose Brown (my nursing classmate in England in 1958), Paula and George Duffy, and Jennifer Copeland, and to my adopted brother, Earle Powell. Thank you all for looking out for me when I am at my home in Florida.

I am forever grateful to my nursing classmates: Betty Lee, RN, BSN, my life coach who has walked me through so many difficult times, and Martha Land, RN, who stood up for me when I became a United States citizen.

Thanks to Nat Wesley of the National Association of Health Services Executives (NAHSE), my friend and advisor on my graduate paper from Johns Hopkins University; Brandon Baptiste (NAHSE) and Darren Brownlee (NAHSE), outstanding young men; Marshall Spurlock, my health and political advisor when I was seeking political office; and Tameka Bell (NAHSE).

My posthumous thanks to Frances Holsey, Bernice Brandford Lewis, Elizabeth Shipley, and Mom Roxie Moore, for being my rock; and to E. Leopold Edwards, my mentor of over fifty years and my reason for running for political office; John (City) Green, my past boss at Lutheran Hospital, later vice president of Medstar Health and friend; Dr. Russell Davis of SHIRE, whom I turned to over the years for his expertise in health care; Maxie Collier, MD, my friend and cofounder of the Black Mental Health Alliance for Education and Consultation; Father Jack Malpas, my first priest who welcomed me to St. Bartholomew's Episcopal Church; Norman Bowmaker, former vice president of Baltimore Gas and Electric who supported all my events; Barbara Kean, my neighbor who invited me to join St. Bartholomew's; Esther McCready, who was able to get Chief Justice Thurgood Marshall to fight for her case to allow Black students to enter the University of Maryland School of Nursing (we became very good friends); Beatrice Reed, the grandmother of comedian Dave Chappelle, who was one of my mentors in the Caribbean American InterCultural Organization (CAIO); and Elijah Saunders, MD, my first cardiologist and friend spanning almost sixty years.

Thanks to Governor Wes Moore, whom I have been so proud of for his warmth, for his charisma, and for caring about people. Most recently, I received from Coppin State University an Honorary Doctorate in Humane Letters in 2021 and an Honorary Doctorate in Public Service from the University of Maryland in 2023.

I am indebted to many organizations I was part of and served as a regular past, active, or honorary member: House of Ruth Maryland; Planned Parenthood of Maryland; National Political Congress of Black Women; Black Congress on Health, Law and Economics (BCHLE); Maryland Black Congress on Health, Law, and Economics (MBCHLE); Chi Eta Phi Sorority; Sigma Theta Tau International Honor Society (inducted at JHU); CAIO; national and local chapters of the Black Nurses Association; American Nurses Association; Maryland Nurses Association; Black Mental Health Alliance for Education and Consultation; Jamaican Association of Maryland (JAM); American Academy of Nursing (fellow); National Black Caucus of State Legislators (NBCSL); National Caucus of State Legislators (NCSL); Maryland Black Caucus of State Legislators (MBCSL); Women Legislators of Maryland; Congress on Health and Economic Disparities (CHED); Congressional Black Caucus Health Brain Trust (CBCHBT); Baltimore City Community College (alumnae); University of Maryland School of Nursing (alumnae); and Johns Hopkins Carey School of Business (alumnae).

SAVING STELLA

Meeting Stella

Call her Stella. She's sitting in a hospital bed in Baltimore. Her dislocated and fractured arm rests in a sling, immobilized. Her injury is a compound fracture, and I am mainly concerned with two things: healing the broken bone and minimizing the risk of infection where the bone has pierced the skin. The smell of antiseptic and hospital-issue soap is strong. I'm moving carefully, bathing her body, dipping the washcloth into the basin, making every attempt not to jar her arm. This isn't part of my usual duties as a team leader, but the hospital is short-staffed and I'm filling in, helping where I can.

Stella is about fifty-five years old, nearly twenty-two years older than I am. She sits, partially covered by a hospital gown, vulnerable, completely dependent on me, her nurse, and others for help with the basic cleansing of her body, something she has handled for most of her life. I lift her arm to wash her armpit. That's when I feel it. Her breast is as hard as a stone.

"How long has your breast been like this?" My voice is steady, strong, giving away nothing. I have learned how to probe without alarming my patients, knowing when to push, when to pull back.

"For quite some time," she says.

From the feel of it, I already know that the solid tissue isn't new and that she has been hiding this for a long time.

"I had no health insurance," she says. "I was waiting to get a job to deal with it."

Stella had recently begun a job driving a school bus when she had the car accident that brought her to the emergency room and, later, to my floor. She had been waiting for some time to secure a job with health benefits and an opportunity to build savings that would allow her to see to the problem with her breast. But that wait could cost her life.

This is not the time to hold back. "You know I have to call the doctor."

"No. Please, no." She looks up at me, her eyes pleading, the desperation in her voice raw.

"I have to. The compound fracture is not what is important now. It is your breast." I already fear the worst.

The doctor comes, and throughout his examination I return to one thought: This patient came through the emergency room and had a cast put on to reset the broken bone, but no one had examined her. How could they have missed a breast as hard as hers?

The missed opportunities to catch the growing lump in her breast stay with me, and later at the nurse's station, I say to the other nurses, "There ought to be a law. There's no reason this woman should be in this condition."

What also stays with me is the fact that having health insurance and obtaining medical care are dependent on one's employment status. The employed have health insurance. The unemployed don't. I came of age in England, and the universal health care system was what I knew. The UK's National Health Service, funded through payroll taxes, guarantees health care for all and provides free health care services—ambulance rides, emergency room visits, radiation, chemotherapy, surgeries, hospitalizations. Stella's situation was surprising, a disappointment for an immigrant like me who had long viewed America as the land where everyone prospered. But I learned early that if your skin is Black or brown and you are poor, America is not always the land of opportunity.

Stella loses the first breast to a mastectomy, loses the second to another mastectomy, loses her hair and stamina to chemotherapy drugs and radiation. When she leaves the hospital, we keep in touch and

I see her a few times through the course of her treatment. Less than two years after our first encounter in the Baltimore hospital, the cancer does indeed take Stella's life.

•

Meeting Stella in 1972 was a pivotal moment in my career. From then on, I knew two truths: nurses must advocate on behalf of their patients, and access to quality health care should be protected by law. I didn't consciously decide to run for office then, but I knew I would fight for improved health care for underserved communities and push for meaningful change for others like Stella. But I didn't do it then. I went to college, earned associate's, bachelor's, and master's degrees, became a quality assurance coordinator, started raising a family, divorced my husband Bill, and finished raising my family as a single parent.

It would take me twenty-five years to honor Stella's memory in a meaningful way. In 1994, I was first elected to the Maryland House of Delegates, and in 1998, my second term in office, I saw one of my early bills passed. The bill provided $2.6 million annually for the diagnosis and treatment of breast cancer in women whose income fell below 250 percent of the federal poverty level. I didn't know then how far Stella's story would take me, or where, or how personal this quest to reduce health care disparities and improve the lives for Black and brown Americans, the underrepresented and the underserved, would become.

In retrospect, it is easy to see how a life takes shape, how a person's calling evolves and manifests. It is easy to draw a line from nursing to managing the circumstances that can affect a person's health—environmental, financial, social—to legislating around those concerns. When I was first elected in 1994, I didn't yet know how my encounters, as a nurse attending to patients in hospitals and as a businesswoman running a personal care company, would influence the bills I sponsored as a member of Maryland's General Assembly. But time after time, I pulled from the well of my experiences as a nurse to effect meaningful change.

PART I

THE EARLY YEARS

CHAPTER 1

My First Life

Finding My Calling

Coming to America was the beginning of my third life. Jamaica is the place of my first life, and England the place of my second. Despite my early reservations about America as a place where I, a Black woman, could thrive, America has proved to be the place where I truly came into my own.

My first concrete understanding of America was as a place that offered promise and opportunity. It was an idea honed by Papa's stories about his time there as a farm worker, stories from relatives who had migrated to America and come back home to Jamaica, as well as general talk about America's greatness that we heard on the radio and read about in magazines, in the *Jamaica Gleaner*, and in books.

My second understanding was characterized by fear of the country and fear for people who looked like me. It was August 1955, and a fourteen-year-old Emmett Till, just two years younger than me, had been killed while visiting family in Mississippi. Those days, I was a young, carefree teen, hiking with friends, spending time at the beach, taking in movies and rock and roll—Bill Haley & His Comets and Elvis Presley. I knew nothing about Mississippi and couldn't imagine the river that gave the state its name. I learned to spell Mississippi from numerous articles in the *Jamaica Gleaner* that carried Till's story. Each new detail about his death haunted me. America was not a place where I wanted to live.

But my sense of America shifted again when I met Bill Pulliam—a soldier in the United States Air Force—at a party in Yorkshire, England, in 1958, a few months after I had arrived in York to study at Bootham Park Hospital School of Nursing. Not long after I met Bill, I knew I was willing to take a gamble and come with him to America if he asked. And my feelings about America as a place of hope and a place full of opportunities for me as a young Black woman strengthened even more in 1960. I was entranced by John F. Kennedy's presidential campaign. After classes, I ran back to the dorms to catch up on the day's developments, and, with his campaign gaining ground, I thought, "Perhaps I can live there." For the first time, I began to see America as it was described by many: the land of opportunity. That hopefulness stayed with me and was part of my worldview when I came to America in November 1960 to join my then husband, Bill.

That belief—seeing America as the land of opportunity—is the one that lasts. It is the one that was part of my consciousness when I met Stella in 1972. But over the years that sense of hope has waxed and waned, particularly when I look at how much work still needs to be done to remove the racial disparities that linger almost everywhere I look.

•

I was born in the district of Waldensia, a rural place in the parish of Trelawny that sits on the edge of Jamaica's Cockpit Country—a rugged limestone plateau in the island's central western region. Waldensia borders Sherwood Content, best known as the hometown of Olympic gold medalist and global sports icon Usain Bolt. The entire district of Waldensia—which comprises Sherwood Content and Greys Inn, where my father, Horace, was born and remained through his early adult years—is a quiet, simple place bordered on the south by the cockpits, thousands of conical hills divided by precipitous ravines. The hills and ravines together form an inhospitable place that sheltered groups of enslaved Africans who fled the plantations and fought for decades to undermine institutionalized slavery. And to the north is the Martha Brae River, which begins somewhere in the cockpits and empties into the sea in the coastal town of Falmouth. To the northwest is Montego Bay, the city that draws many of the area's residents.

My mother, a dressmaker, whom everyone called Miss Beauty, was one of those people in search of a better life. She moved to Montego Bay, leaving me in Greys Inn with Papa, a carpenter who worked for the Department of Public Works.

When I was three years old, Papa got a job in Panama. He sent word to my mother that he would bring me to live with her. We went by bus, moving along the coast, through Falmouth and Greenwood and Rose Hall, past the plot of land that would later become the site of the Donald Sangster International Airport and on into the city proper. Montego Bay was very different from Greys Inn, where I had acres of land to run around and two grandfathers who lived nearby.

We stood outside the house where Mama lived, waiting for her to come home. Though she expected us, she was late returning from work. Papa had to catch a bus back to Greys Inn. He was leaving for Panama the following day. He paced back and forth outside the house, nervous and watchful.

The woman I would call Aunt Lize stepped out. She was a slim, dark-skinned woman with a beautiful smile. Aunt Lize volunteered to watch me until my mother came home. Papa stooped and said his good-byes. His leaving was then the greatest loss of my life. I cried when he left; until then, he was the only parent I had known. When he was gone, I stayed outside at the top of a stairway, teary-eyed, comforted for a time by a senseh fowl—a common chicken without feathers in its midsection—that Aunt Lize gave me to pet.

My mother, Miss Beauty, cried when she saw me. This was her first time seeing me in a couple of years. She also cried because she didn't know who would watch me when she went to work.

"Miss Beauty, don't worry," Aunt Lize said. "I will take care of Shirley."

That first Monday, Mama enrolled me in school—a new experience for me. Roll call was among the first items of the day, and when the teacher called my name, I ran from the classroom, past the other children, away from the two-story schoolhouse, around the corner to home. Luckily, Aunt Lize was there, and she took me back to school. That time I stayed.

I remember very little about my early days. Some details are clear. We moved to Barnett Street when I was five, and we were close enough that I could walk to the nearby Barracks Road School. I remember that England, Jamaica's mother country, was still fighting World War II. One night, the police came to the door, knocking loudly and shouting orders to turn off the lights so enemy bombers wouldn't see any potential targets. Scared, I pulled the covers over my head. I remember the after-school games we children played, parading in the yard like market women, with baskets on our heads. Sometimes we'd fill the baskets with stones, and once, the heavy basket fell from my head and the large stone in it crushed my left big toe. I screamed and hobbled home. My toe was bleeding so badly Mama rushed me off to the hospital. But we were not daunted by injuries like those.

We performed weddings and funerals for any insect or animal that died. Many years after I had moved from Montego Bay and after a three-month hospital stay for rheumatic fever, I performed the biggest funeral for my parrot, Pretty, a gift from Papa, who chirped my name and woke me up for school in the mornings. I was quite attached to Pretty, and before going to the hospital, I asked my Aunt Vera to take care of the bird and make sure it had its usual diet of peppers, corn, and water. Finally discharged after so many months, and home just in time to celebrate my tenth birthday, I was excited to see Pretty again. I hurried to its cage, said, "Hi, Pretty," and scratched its head. The parrot turned around and died.

Tears welled up. I was devastated by the sudden loss. It seemed that during my hospitalization, no one had fed the bird and it lived just long enough to greet me. I buried Pretty with buttercups on her grave and we sang the hymn "Abide with Me."

One day, years before, while I was playing outside in my bare feet, a woman stopped and introduced herself as Miss Plummer. I would come to call her Aunt Vera. Mama wasn't home, but Aunt Vera said my father had told her that he had a little girl named Shirley. Aunt Vera had come to see me and to ask my mother if I could spend some time with her in Kingston, Jamaica's capital city. I ran inside, told our helper I had to go with the visitor to get Mama, put my shoes on, and accompanied Aunt Vera to the market, where Mama owned a stall from which she sold the clothes she made. Later, she worked as a buyer and a manager for two prominent department stores in Montego Bay. Mama and Aunt Vera liked each other, and about a month later, I went to visit Aunt Vera.

For my first trip to Kingston, which is on the eastern end of the island, I traveled alone by train. Mama put me in a seat by the window so I could look out and asked the conductor to look after me. It was not unusual for strangers to look after a child traveling alone, and the other passengers on the train made sure I didn't go hungry, sharing with me oranges and cashews and dried shrimp that vendors sold at various train stops, even though Mama had packed my lunch. I was a picky eater. When I was younger, my grandfather, having seen me give my food to the dogs under the table, would pick sour oranges, roast them, and sprinkle the slices with sugar to increase my appetite. On the train, however, I ate the food the strangers offered.

That first evening at Aunt Vera's house, which was across the street from the restaurant she owned, I sat on a stool swinging my legs when a man came and stood before me. I thought nothing of his presence, thought nothing of him asking my name.

"Little girl, are you waiting for someone?" he asked.

"Yes, my father is coming to see me this evening."

"Would you recognize him?"

"Yes, he's missing the first inch of his little finger." I reached out to show him where the finger was missing a piece and saw the shortened finger. I screamed, "Papa!"

My father left for America to be a farmworker when I was four years old. So I really forgot what his face actually looked like. When he had returned to Jamaica, he had moved to Kingston and was living there with his new family.

After that first summer visit, I went back to Montego Bay, but when I was about seven years old, Papa and Aunt Vera decided I should return to Kingston, where Aunt Vera enrolled me in Mico Practicing School. Papa introduced me to my sister Valerie, already a year old. Valerie was the best sight I'd ever seen. I had been longing for a sister, and there she was: a crying baby in diapers just learning to walk. My stepmother, Mae, had another child, Harlene—a chubby newborn girl.

I stayed on with Aunt Vera, living with her as if I were her own child, even spending the summer months with her parents in Catadupa, a small town in the parish of St. James on the western edge of Cockpit Country. Both of my grandmothers, Emily and Maryann, had died before I was born. Papa's father, whom everyone called Mas Nick, died at the age of ninety-two, when I was nine, and I remember the trip back to Greys Inn for his funeral.

When we arrived in town, I heard people saying, "Mas Nick look so good." Hearing that, I thought he was alive and well, and I was upset when I got to the house and saw him laid out on the bed dressed in his suit. Papa and some men from the neighborhood cut down a mahogany tree to make Mas Nick's casket. After the casket was lined, I playfully climbed into it. But Papa quickly removed me. Rain poured throughout the funeral, and water filled the grave. As his casket was lowered into the ground, I worried he was going to drown. That day was the first time I saw Papa cry. I looked closely, thinking it was simply rainwater on his face, realizing soon that Papa was crying for his father.

On another visit back to my parents' hometown in Trelawny, I visited Mama's father, Joseph Calomathi, whom we called Mas Joe. On one of those visits, Mama "kidnapped" my older brother, Lloyd, who was living in Sherwood Content with family. I was about five and Lloyd about eight. We spent our days playing with our aunt and uncle, Verna and Alfred, who were about the same age as we were. Mas Joe had remarried after my grandmother's death and started a new family.

Rain poured the day we got ready to leave. Mama slipped Lloyd into the back of the truck and covered him with a tarpaulin. Mama and I sat in the front of the truck. But the passenger side had no door and rain poured in on us. I was scared we would fall out. But I was more worried about Lloyd covered under the tarpaulin in the back.

"Lloyd's going to drown," I said.

Mama hushed me and said Lloyd would be okay. When we were a little ways out of town, she asked someone to send word back to her family that Lloyd was with her.

•

When I was about seven years old, I discovered something about myself: I couldn't tell time. Also, I couldn't tell *b* from *d*, or *m* from *n*, and sounding out letters was difficult. I spelled my name *Mathan* instead of *Nathan*, frustrating Papa to no end. Math was especially challenging because I reversed numbers. Standing at the blackboard in front of my classmates crushed me. I never answered the problems correctly. I sat in the back, hoping my teachers didn't call on me and hiding my frustration.

A few years later, I heard my parents discussing my learning difficulties. Mama decided to have me tutored. My parents didn't know anything about dyslexia—a learning disability that makes it difficult to read, write, and spell. It would be years before I, too, learned that word and some coping strategies. But the one-on-one tutoring saved my educational life. My tutor was a retired teacher, Mrs. Wright, who had taught my older brother math in Montego Bay. After she retired, she moved to Kingston.

Later, when I was about thirteen, she asked a group of students, "You know whose sister that is?"

The other students couldn't guess. Mrs. Wright answered her own question by calling my brother's name, Lloyd, although those children did not know him. Lloyd had always excelled at mathematics, and I couldn't measure up to the standard he had set. I struggled on, disappointing Papa time and time again. In addition, when I entered puberty, I began experiencing classic migraines with aura and nausea and had to stay in bed in a dark room. I lost many school days because of the migraines.

I was anxious. What would become of me? My anxiety increased even more when, at thirteen, I went to live with my father and step-mother. Aunt Vera, busy with running a restaurant, couldn't keep track of me all the time. Many times, I told her I was going around the corner, and instead, I would be miles away. Papa decided I would come to live with him, my stepmother, and my four siblings.

Moving to Papa's house brought its own set of challenges. I was expected to help with my younger siblings and do housework, something I hadn't done while living with Aunt Vera since she had helpers who took care of such chores. And now Papa had a direct line to my academic progress.

"You're going to end up cleaning houses." That's the refrain from my childhood. Its echo hurts me, even now. I hear Papa telling me, in front of my siblings, that I was dumb and would amount to nothing. Many times at the dining table he ordered my younger sister and brother, "Tell Shirley what seven times four is." He knew I couldn't give him the answer. Embarrassed, I dreaded those meals.

At other moments, though, I was on top of the world. I joined everything: Brownies, 4-H Club, Junior Red Cross Society, and Junior Daughters of the King—an order in the Anglican Church—at St. Luke's Anglican Church in the Cross Roads section of Kingston, the same church where I was confirmed at age twelve. I was an active member of the Girl Guides Association, the equivalent of the Girl Scouts. When King George VI died in 1952, I was tasked with lowering the flag at the Girl Guides Headquarters in Kingston. And later, I had the job of hoisting the flag for the services in Jamaica marking the coronation of Queen Elizabeth II.

Outside of Girl Guides, I was failing at everything. My siblings excelled at academics and went to prestigious high schools—Holy Childhood High School, Excelsior High School, Calabar High School, and Wolmer's Boys School. I, on the other hand, had a short-lived stint at a dressmaking shop. I love being around people, and dressmaking, with its hours of concentrating on small needles and thread and various types of stitches, wasn't for me. I wanted to engage and interact with people, and I knew early on that I had to find something else.

Luckily, when I was about to turn seventeen, Mama sent for me. I returned to Montego Bay and got my first job working with Dr. Herbert Morrison and my cousin, Dr. Noel Black, in their medical practice. Later Dr. Warren Wilson, a surgeon, joined the practice. I did everything, from handling urine tests to drawing blood to assisting with minor surgeries and making house calls.

The job confirmed what I had known to be my calling since I was nine years old, when I was hospitalized at the Kingston Public Hospital (KPH) for three months with rheumatic fever. The infection started, I believe, one afternoon when I was walking home from school in a heavy thunderstorm. The gutters were overflowing with water. The other students and I took off our shoes and jumped up and down in the rainwater flowing through the gutters. That evening, I could not swallow, my throat was sore, and my tonsils were swollen. Aunt Vera and I thought it was just a cold. But my fever kept going up. Aunt Vera took me to see a doctor on Duke Street, who put me on a medication that tasted of wintergreen. But that didn't work. My feet started to swell and I couldn't walk. The adults around me had to lift and carry me from place to place. Clearly whatever was wrong was more serious than a cold, and I was admitted to the hospital and diagnosed with rheumatic fever.

During those three months, I got to know the nurses really well, and I discovered that the nurses who came on shift in the morning read the doctors' notes. They knew I had to stay in bed on bed rest. But the nurses who came in the afternoon didn't read the notes, which made it possible for me to make rounds with them. I saw all the patients, helped with bedpans, fetched water, and shared my food with them.

My case of rheumatic fever affected my heart, causing systolic heart murmurs. I was brought by wheelchair into a room full of doctors who were discussing my case. Unsure if I would live or die, they decided I should stay on the adult ward.

One morning I began wrapping my doll the way the staff wrapped the patients who had died. My doctor, seeing me, said, "It's time to send Shirley home."

I'd had a taste of caring for patients and knew that was what I wanted to do. I wanted to be just like those nurses who took care of me, and I never changed my mind.

Not long into my job in the doctor's office, I decided to go to nursing school. Because of my learning difficulties, I was concerned I wouldn't be able to pass the entry exams at the university level. I explored training programs at hospitals, including KPH, but KPH had a long wait list. So I looked for programs outside of Jamaica and found a nursing program in York, England. I wrote a letter requesting an application. When the letter arrived, I applied right away, and was thrilled when I heard that the program had accepted me.

But getting to York wasn't easy. Papa refused to help with the money I needed to travel to England, telling me that I had to prove to him that I could do it, just as he had to prove himself to his father.

When Papa decided he wanted to learn carpentry, his father gave him a hammer and all the tools he needed, and said that as soon as he could afford to buy his own he should return the ones he was given. When Papa received his first paycheck, he bought his own set of tools and returned everything his father had given him.

I was determined to go. I saved every penny I made and joined a partner—an informal, cooperative saving system that is popular in Jamaica. Each member of the group deposits a fixed sum to the banker or treasurer weekly (or whatever schedule the group determines). Each week, the banker pays out the hand—the full amount collected—to a member in rotation until everyone in the group receives a draw. It was a quick way of saving a lump sum.

The day I went to pick up my passport in Kingston, I wore an A-line turquoise dress with a black-and-white kick at the bottom. Wanting to show my father what I had accomplished, I went to his job site. He was working as a contractor and builder then, building a school near Mountain View Avenue.

"Where you going dress up so?" he asked.

"I went to pick up my passport," I said. "I'm going to England."

Papa smiled. He was proud. I had aced his test.

"How much did you spend on the airfare?" he asked.

When I told him the amount, he reached into his pocket and gave me back what I had spent.

In the midst of my preparations to leave, Mama became ill with pneumonia. I had to shift my priorities to take care of her. The doctors didn't think she would make it. She was hospitalized and unconscious. With treatment options exhausted, the doctors decided to administer ampicillin, an antibiotic newly available in the Caribbean. Ampicillin, which was already in use in other developed countries, was so new that the hospital did not yet have it in stock. I had to purchase it at an off-site pharmacy and bring it in. That treatment worked, and Mama began to improve.

When she woke up, she called me "Clara," her sister's name. With tears in my eyes, I told her it was me, Shirley. She told me about her dream: She was on one side of a river and on the other side were her father and deceased siblings—Lucille, a nurse who had died before I was born, and her brother Melvin, who had been a police officer. Mama wanted to get across the river to meet them and reached out her hand. But the three of them said, "No, Beauty. We aren't ready for you to come as yet."

With Mama out of the hospital and recuperating, I resumed planning my departure. I visited friends and family, bringing an autograph book and asking everyone to write inspirational quotes. All the quotes were special to me, but three have remained with me all these years. They are words I live by:

I wish thee neither riches nor the glow of greatness but that wherever you go some weary heart may gladden at your smile, some weary heart know sunshine for a while, so that thy days shall be a track of light, like angels' footsteps in the passing night.

People who care about others give the world its real beauty and life its true meaning.

And I said to the man who stood at the gate of the year: "Give me a light that I may tread safely into the unknown." And he replied: "Go out into the darkness and put your hand into the Hand of God. That shall be to you better than light and safer than a known way."

I left Jamaica on a clear day in August 1958. Mama, Papa, my stepmother, my sister Valerie, and my brothers Nicholas and Errol came to the airport to see me off. My sister, Harlene, who was living in Montego Bay with her aunt at that time, wasn't able to make it.

"Shirley, are you coming back tomorrow?" asked Errol, my youngest brother, with tears in his eyes.

"No, Errol, not tomorrow. But you'll hear from me," I said and gave him a big hug.

"Beauty," Papa said. "You and I didn't make it, but our daughter didn't turn out so bad after all." I sensed his pride in what I had accomplished. His approval meant the world to me.

It was time to go. I hugged my family one last time, wiping away tears as I walked away. As the plane taxied down the runway and began to lift off, I peered out the window, trying to catch a last glimpse of my family waving at the rising, roaring plane. Looking down on the island, I saw with clarity what my Uncle Roland had told me. As he was preparing to write his quote in my autograph book, he'd said, "You are on your own, Shirley. You have to think about that. There's no family to take care of you."

CHAPTER 2

Going to England

Shannon, a town on Ireland's west coast, was the first stop on my flight to York, England, and I had my first taste of the cold and dreary weather for which that region is known. We were there for several hours, but I didn't get a chance to travel through the city. Even though it was August, I was grateful for my warm coat and boots, which I had purchased from a Jamaican woman who had lived in England and returned home. We flew on to London, and after I cleared customs I took a taxi to the train station where I boarded the train for York.

All my life, I had heard about London, and there it was—sunny and not particularly gloomy that day. Its brick buildings quickly slipped by the train windows, and I peered out trying to catch a glimpse of the place that left a mark on Jamaica and several other Caribbean islands. Jamaica would remain a British colony until 1962 when it became an independent, self-governing nation.

Three hours later I was in York, standing outside the wrought iron gates of the Bootham Park Hospital with two big suitcases. Though the school had instructed me to take a taxi from the train station to the campus, two women I befriended on the train assured me that I could take the bus directly there. I had followed their advice, realizing too late that while the bus did, indeed, stop at the hospital, the campus itself was vast and the distance from the gate to the nurse's residence too great a distance for me to walk with my two large suitcases. I waved down a taxi as I should have done from the outset.

The campus was beautiful, with trees and flowers lining the long driveway. As the taxi made its way across the grounds, I took in the red brick buildings, the architecture so unlike what I was accustomed to in Jamaica. At last I made it to the nurse's residence, which was to the right of the hospital. I was greeted by the housemother, who showed me to my room. I was excited to learn that there were twelve other Jamaican young women in the nursing program.

The food, however, was bland and missing all the spices I had grown up knowing. Neither I nor the other Jamaican women ate the food. And, like I always do, I made friends quickly, this time with the gardener who gave me cabbage and onions, and also with a cook in the kitchen who gave me bacon. One of the older students, Icy McDonald, already a married woman, chopped up the cabbage and onions and sautéed them with the bacon, making meals for all of us and later teaching me how to cook. I had managed to get through my teen years without having learned because Aunt Vera had household help who cooked and cleaned. When I went to live with my father, I had to help my stepmother with cleaning but I was too young to cook. Later, when I returned to Montego Bay to live with Mama, she also had helpers, so again I did not have to cook. I was grateful to Icy for teaching me how to make basic meals.

That first winter and every one after I missed Jamaica fiercely. I missed hearing the birds singing and stepping outside into the full, warm sunshine. The dreary, dull, and foggy weather was depressing. One of my greatest challenges was walking to classes in the snow and fog. At first I loved the novelty of snow, but I quickly came to see the challenges of walking in it. Getting to classes meant we had to cross a busy street near the Rowntree Chocolate Factory. Most of the Rowntree employees rode bicycles to work, and trying to get to classes in the morning was a dangerous escapade. Imagine standing at the crosswalk in thick fog and seeing nothing but bicycles on the road coming toward you. With the fog, it was difficult to see, and getting across the street was like taking our lives into our hands.

But when spring arrived, the vivid yellow, bright purple, and deep red flowers transformed the land into a beautiful and different place. The transformation was breathtaking, and the renewed sense of life reinvigorated me too.

·

I met Bill one Christmas. I was nineteen years old, still living in the dorms at Bootham Park Hospital. A group of friends attending nearby St. John's College—all immigrants from West Africa, mainly Nigeria, Ghana, and Sierra Leone—hosted a party in a hotel. The girls in the group gave me African attire to wear, taught me a greeting in Swahili, and asked me to greet visitors as they came in. Not until later in the evening did I learn that what they taught me was no greeting. All evening I had been greeting the men with "I want to love you." Fending off the men who took my misspoken greeting seriously was a task.

Halfway through the evening, I opened the door to a tall, dark-skinned young man.

"Can I come into the party?" he asked.

I let him in. Since the hosts were all from various countries in Africa, I thought he was as well. "What part of Africa are you from?" I asked.

"Pardon me, miss, I am from the USA," he said.

Bill was in the Air Force, the 47th Bomb Squad, and was staying in the hotel for a few days. He was stationed in Leeds and had come to York to say goodbye to a girl he was dating. We talked, danced to Paul Anka's "Diana," and took pictures. Before I knew it, I had stayed longer than I should have. By the time my girlfriends, Norma and Clemmy, and I returned to the dorms, it was past curfew, and the only way to get back in without being seen was climbing through the coal closet in my white chiffon, embroidered dress. We had to return before bed check or else the party we had been planning for the following day would have been canceled. We made our way through the coal closet as quietly and quickly as we could. Luckily, we got back just in time.

Before I left the party, I invited Bill to the party we were hosting the day after Christmas, which is celebrated in British Commonwealth countries as Boxing Day. Bill came, along with two fellow GIs. We corresponded by mail, and I saw Bill again for his birthday. Then he was sent to Germany, and I didn't hear from him for a while. Thinking he was no longer interested, I began dating another man, a Jamaican named Winston.

Six months later, I received a letter from Bill asking me to marry him. I was torn, excited by Bill's accent and the differences between our cultures, but comforted by the culture I shared with Winston. This was a very stressful time for me, trying to decide which of the two men to marry. I even wrote to Dear Abby for help. Winston was planning to take me to Manchester to meet his mother and sister. After a shopping trip to find shoes that would not make me appear taller than Winston, I broke it off. He did not take it lightly.

The simple truth was that I was more attracted to Bill, and I wanted to marry him. Before the wedding, I had to go to the Air Force base in Norfolk to fill out immigration forms and undergo counseling and a physical. Mama had asked a few questions and readily gave her blessing, but my father was not happy. I assumed he wanted me to practice nursing in Jamaica. And he may have been looking forward to giving me away.

One month after my twenty-first birthday, I married Bill, surrounded by my nursing school classmates, my professor, my cousin Cherry from London, and Jean Paul Roperio, who acted as my giveaway father. While I was in living in York, Jean Paul, a French man, and his English wife, Eileen, had become my surrogate parents. My nursing school classmates served as my bridesmaids and Cherry was my chief bridesmaid. The children of another cousin, Bunny, were the flower girls. My parents were not there, but Mama was there in spirit through the four-tier lace and chiffon bridal gown she had made and sent to me in England. We were married at St. Mary's Anglican Church, which is located near the famous York Minster. The church was decorated with pink rosebuds lining the altar and aisle. I carried pink rosebuds as my bouquet, and my headdress was covered with orange blossoms. It was a beautiful ceremony on a bright and sunny day— a rarity in York's normally gloomy weather. This moment marked a transition to a life I had never imagined as a girl growing up in Jamaica, particularly a dyslexic girl who had been told time and time again that she would not excel.

Bill and I spent our honeymoon in London, walking through Hyde Park, looking at all the sites, and enjoying different aspects of English life. We also visited family in London and then returned to Yorkshire.

My time in England came to an end not long after our wedding. Bill was discharged from the Air Force in September 1960 and subsequently went to Baltimore, where his parents and siblings had settled after moving from North Carolina. Before he left we made plans for me to join him there soon after, and I set about packing up my life and getting ready to start anew in another country.

What did I know about America? What kind of a life was I running toward?

The 1960 election campaign was underway. John F. Kennedy was the candidate I had been watching from afar. Kennedy was young, confident, energetic, and progressive, and as I prepared to leave England and move to America, I paid closer attention to his campaign and his promises, as well as the continuing fight for civil rights. There was no forgetting that Emmett Till had been murdered just five years earlier simply because of the color of his skin, no way to ignore the protests and sit-ins that were becoming a regular part of the struggle for civil rights, the violence, and the arrests. In the weeks leading up to the election, Dr. Martin Luther King Jr. was arrested during a protest in Atlanta, Georgia.

Much later I would learn about the Greensboro sit-in that started in 1960 after young African American students sat at a segregated Woolworths lunch counter in Greensboro, North Carolina, and refused to leave after being denied service. Not long after, the sit-in as a form of protest spread to college towns across the southern states. The students were beaten and arrested, but the protests continued and forced

Woolworths and other establishments to change their policies. And in Baltimore, students at Morgan State University used the same approach to force the Read's Drug Store chain to desegregate. But I didn't know then about these protests so close to the place that would become my home.

In the fall months before I arrived in America, I went to the nursing lounge after classes to watch the day's roundup of the campaign activities, Kennedy's movement across the country, and Dr. King's endorsement of Kennedy. When Kennedy won in November, I was elated. I had high expectations about what he could accomplish and how he could expand civil rights for Black people in America. His win, I hoped, was the start of a new era.

CHAPTER 3

Coming to America

I arrived in New York from England on a cold November day in 1960 after a ten-hour flight. My feet were swollen, my belly rounded. I was six and a half months pregnant. Because of excessive weight gain, I was uncomfortable, cold, and anxious, simply miserable. The small, cramped plane didn't help. Bill, his mother, Annie, and a friend, Albert, came to meet me at the airport. Everything was new—America, my marriage, Bill's family, and Bill's post-service career.

What I thought would be about a thirty-minute ride home turned out to be a four-hour-long trip from New York City, through New Jersey and Delaware and the northern reaches of Maryland. We drove through Baltimore, past some beautiful homes with wide porches and verandas, and I expected that at any minute we would stop at one of them. But when the car finally stopped, we were in front of a three-story, stone building—a tenement house on Linden Avenue in West Baltimore.

In York, after I had moved out of the dormitory, I shared a flat with a classmate. We had two large bedrooms, a living room, a dining room, and a kitchen. Except for the lack of central heating—we had fireplaces and slept with hot water bottles tucked into our sheets—the flat was perfect. What I found in Baltimore was not perfect by any means. My in-laws—Bill's parents—his two sisters, and his two brothers lived in a first-floor apartment. His parents had converted the dining room into a bedroom for us. There were no doors—just a curtain hung to give us some semblance of privacy. To get to the bedrooms in the back, the bathroom, or the kitchen, everyone walked through our makeshift bedroom. It was not an ideal living arrangement for newlyweds expecting a baby. Coming from England, where my body had adapted to colder temperatures with no central heating indoors, I found the apartment to be extremely hot, almost unbearable.

But perhaps the biggest shock were the distinct differences between the American medical system and England's socialized medicine program. Under England's socialized medicine program, I, as a pregnant woman, received vitamins, milk, and juice delivered directly to my home each week. And during my pregnancy when I suffered from severe morning sickness (hyperemesis gravidarum), my doctor came to the house to give me IV fluids to prevent dehydration. The doctor was also monitoring my long-standing heart condition (I have had a heart murmur since childhood). The British system was set up to ensure that mothers-to-be have healthy pregnancies. In America, I was largely on my own, fully responsible for buying my own vitamins and other nourishments.

The first order of business was finding a doctor. I decided to register at the University of Maryland Medical Center's Obstetrics Clinic and quickly found that I would not have a private physician. For each visit, I would be seen by any available doctor. In clinics like these, each visit with the doctor meant that I had to spend time telling yet another physician my history. I know now how important continuity of care is to a patient's overall outcome, as well as the trust the patient builds in his or her doctor. But as a young woman and a new immigrant, I had little choice.

Bill didn't have many options regarding work. In the military, he had served as a clerk inputting data, but his skill set was limited, so he went to work in a hospital during the winter months and in construction during the warmer months. He left for work early in the morning, returning home in the late afternoon. His schedule left me alone with his family members, each of whom spoke with a deep Southern accent. His family didn't understand my Jamaican accent and I didn't understand theirs. Where I shortened vowel sounds, Americans stretched them out, and where I lengthened them, Americans shortened. When Bill's friend Albert introduced himself, I heard Abbott, and I called him Abbott for weeks until I saw his written name.

I learned quickly that the differences I admired between Bill's culture and mine were the things that stood between us. My family pushed education as the defining factor that would help me and my siblings move along in the world. Bill, on the other hand, had grown up with a different set of priorities. In North Carolina, they had been sharecroppers. That exploitative system meant day-to-day survival was their top concern. Bill and his family had worked hard picking tobacco and cotton, working all hours and weekends in the southern heat to maintain the quota of crops mandated by the landowner and to ensure they could pay the landowner his share of the crops they reaped and the rent for the house on that same property, in which they lived. Our childhood experiences were markedly different. Mine was more carefree. I was free on weekends to see movies at the cinema. Bill had to work with his family in the fields and wasn't able to do some of the things I did. Newly arrived in Baltimore, Bill's family was still trying to make a steady life. In Jamaica, I was used to sitting down together as a family to eat dinner and have conversations. In Baltimore, each member of Bill's family ate as he or she arrived home. There was a lot to adjust to in my new life.

•

Late on a snowy evening in early February—February 2, Groundhog Day—I went into labor. It was a long labor—over twenty-four hours long. Since I was delivering in a teaching hospital, doctor after doctor came to examine me to determine why my labor was lasting so long. I almost lost my mind. Finally, baby Wayne was born on February 3, his father's birthday. At the time, I could not go shopping for a birthday gift for Bill because I did not yet understand dollars and cents; I still calculated everything in British pounds, shillings, and pence. So I looked at the baby boy as Bill's birthday gift.

Change came fast after Wayne was born. Bill, Wayne, and I moved about a mile away to our own apartment on Eutaw Place, a one bedroom with large living and dining rooms. I also decided to get a job. The Maryland Board of Nursing, however, which licenses nurses to work in the state, advised me that they would not accept my certifications from the General Nursing Council for England and Wales. In England, I had specialized in psychiatry and had not taken pediatrics and obstetrics courses. The licensing board encouraged me to go to Baltimore City Hospital and enroll in the licensed practical nurses program, which included obstetrics and pediatrics classes. So I returned to nursing school—the Baltimore City Hospital School of Nursing—to become a licensed practical nurse.

The nursing school was a forty-five-minute bus ride from my home. I changed buses in downtown Baltimore, sometimes in the wee hours of the morning. I was often frightened, walking and standing alone among the tall, gray buildings in that part of town, so lonely, desolate, and unattractive that time of morning. Today this area is the beautiful Inner Harbor, which attracts millions of tourists each year, much changed from the industrial area of the 1960s. Some of those mornings I got turned around and caught the bus going in the wrong direction, still thinking I was in England, where the traffic is on the opposite side of the street. But I persisted and in 1962, I graduated and sat for the State Board of Nurses Exam.

When I started working at Baltimore City Hospital—now called Hopkins Bayview Medical Center—I was assigned to work in a lab to sterilize distilled water and other liquids that are required in the operating room. That was not the job for me. I wanted to work with patients. Three months after I started in that role, I called the Nursing Services Department and told them I would leave if I wasn't allowed to practice nursing. With that one complaint, I was moved into obstetrics and gynecology and the newborn nursery.

Finally, I was on my way to practicing the kind of nursing work I had studied so hard to do. It would be another ten years before my encounter with Stella changed the trajectory of my life, but I was well on my way.

CHAPTER 4

Learning the Modern American View of Race

Understanding Disparities

Some fifty years later, I still remember one patient's words as clear as day. It was morning, and I was making rounds at the hospital in Baltimore—checking in with each patient and recording their status, taking and noting blood sugar and blood pressure readings, looking for issues that required immediate intervention, and dispensing medication. The patient—an older white man, around sixty years old—sat on the edge of the bed, clearly uncomfortable, and when I asked how he was feeling he said he needed an enema. I made a note of it and assured him he would get one that day.

I went about my day, and much later, near the end of my shift, as I walked through his room, he said he hadn't received the enema.

"I gave that order to your nurse this morning," I said, concerned about what else the nursing staff may have missed.

"I couldn't let that dainty, little blue-eyed, blond nurse give me an enema," he said. His voice carried across the room.

I knew exactly what that meant, how he saw me as a Black nurse, what he thought was appropriate for the Black nurse to do. I saw how he compartmentalized my colleague, put her on a pedestal because of the color of her skin, hair, and eyes, and his perception of what her constitution should and shouldn't handle.

But in that moment in the hospital room, I simply said, "Well, this Black girl ain't going to give it to you." It was the end of my shift and

I gave the report to the oncoming nurse, laying out our exact conversation, and asked her to take care of him.

Much later, I saw how the perceptions that male patient held about the constitution of Black and white women played out in the broader world, in patient care, in the inequities that mark Black lives in Baltimore and across America. That encounter wasn't the kind of thing that happened often, but it sits in my mind as a broad example of race in America and the prejudices and assumptions that often follow, as well as what is thought to be appropriate for one race and not for another.

I had heard the N-word before, mostly in the psychiatric unit or coming from irrational and out-of-control patients, those with dementia or hallucinations, or alcoholics in withdrawal. When patients were in that kind of distress, they called the staff all kinds of names. The first time a patient called me the N-word directly I was still in England, treating a psychiatric patient who was in the midst of a breakdown and on a rampage. I didn't take it personally; in Yorkshire, there were few Blacks and I didn't see anybody else being treated unfairly simply because of the color of their skin. I chalked up the slur to the person's mental state and went about my business.

But in Baltimore, I faced a different set of circumstances, which carried America's centuries-long history of segregation. I hadn't encountered that anywhere else. I had come into my twenties and to America without firsthand experience. Not until I went to North Carolina during my first year in America did I come face-to-face with how segregation worked. We were traveling by car to Greensboro—my husband, his parents and sisters, and Wayne. On the highway, the towns flew by—a blur of forests, the occasional farm with cattle and farm equipment, glimpses of towns beyond the highway. We were content in our bubble, laughing and talking, and stopping to eat the fried chicken and biscuits my mother-in-law had prepared. She was a great cook, and we went through the chicken and biscuits fast, faster than we should have. Hungry, I asked Bill to stop for hamburgers. He got out of the car and began walking to the back of the store.

I called him back and asked, "Why are you going around the back?" "Blacks can't go to the front of the store," he said.

Stunned by the requirement that Black patrons enter through the back, I said to Bill, "Please come back in the car. I don't want it."

That hadn't been my experience in Baltimore. I had heard stories, of course, about department stores that didn't allow Black shoppers to try on hats in stores, how retail staff followed Black patrons around but didn't do the same to white patrons. The Read's Drug Store sit-in and related civil rights campaigns orchestrated by students at Morgan State University in the 1950s and 1960s were still ongoing when I arrived in Baltimore. As a new immigrant, I didn't yet know the rules—written or unwritten—for how we navigated each neighborhood, or tried on clothes or shoes. That first year, I had spent the first few months waiting for the birth of my child, and when the baby arrived, I spent most of my days attending to the never-ending needs of a newborn. Besides, I had little money to spend and couldn't afford the department stores around Baltimore. So until that moment, I hadn't felt that I was treated as a second-class citizen. Or perhaps I was too young and naive to see what was happening around me. I was shocked that something as simple as buying food could undermine your sense of self-worth.

Then, I knew why my mother-in-law had cooked, why we carried our own food, and I knew, too, that what felt like a family picnic when we stopped to eat carried a larger weight, a darker message about the country in which we lived.

We carried on to Greensboro, a country town where Bill's family had a large house with several bedrooms. But the house had no indoor toilet. While there was a makeshift shower outside, we had to go to the bushes to relieve ourselves. While urban areas across America had long had running water and electricity, indoor plumbing and electricity came to many rural communities late, and this rural part of Greensboro hadn't yet moved forward with the times. This was new, another shock. Even in the most rural areas in Jamaica, a house without indoor plumbing had a pit toilet or latrine at the very least.

Again, I found myself thinking that the wealthiest country in the world was failing some of its residents.

•

By the time I moved to Baltimore in 1960, Verda Welcome, an African American teacher and civil rights leader, had been a member of the Maryland House of Delegates for two years, representing what was then Baltimore's Fourth District. In 1962, she was elected to the Maryland State Senate and served for two decades, becoming the first Black person elected to the senate of Maryland. Years later, when I first ran for an elected office, Verda Welcome was the first elected person to contribute to my campaign. And it was a tremendous honor to find myself as a newly elected senator in 2014 sitting in the same state senate chamber where she had served. She would have been proud.

Having a Black woman in the Maryland House of Delegates in 1960 was a significant achievement. It wasn't until 1968 that Shirley Chisholm became the first African American woman elected to the United States Congress. But the system and policies that had historically prevented Black people from advancing had lingering effects, and the majority of Blacks in Baltimore were struggling to survive. In 1960, the white population in Baltimore City was 610,608, while the Black population was just about half at 325,589. In the decade before I came to Baltimore, median earnings for households in Baltimore City and nearby suburban households were about the same. But as more affluent households began moving to the suburbs, the number of poor residents in the city increased.[1]

Where Bill and I lived, most of the people around us were poor, and only a small percentage held professional jobs. Census data shows that in 1960, a little over 52,000 whites and 7,700 Blacks in Baltimore were employed in professional and technical, and managerial and proprietary, fields.[2] In Jamaica, I had grown up with people who looked like me serving as doctors, firefighters, and police officers. One of my uncles had served as the assistant chief of firefighters in Montego Bay, and

I spent many an afternoon sliding down the pole in the firehouse where he worked. In Baltimore I saw a different set of circumstances. There were few Blacks in the police force and few who were firefighters. By 1965, though, more opportunities for Blacks opened up as the system and policies that had historically prevented Blacks from advancing through these careers were beginning to change slowly.

Throughout the early sixties, the Black population in West Baltimore increased, and as it did, white families sold their properties, sometimes well below market rate, and moved to the suburbs.[3] Bill and I also moved, but for different reasons. The community we chose, the Hunting Ridge community above Edmondson Village, was beautiful at that time and the crime rate low, with a mixture of large single-family homes, duplexes, and row houses set amid tall and mature trees. We liked it because most everything was within walking distance—grocery stores, bakeries, banks, a movie theater, the elementary school, and large department stores. Living in a walkable neighborhood was important because we had only one car.

We moved in the spring of 1966 and unknowingly integrated a street. I sensed that I was being watched, and I could see eyes peeping through the curtains and blinds. When I looked, the person peeping out moved away. There was an undercurrent of tension in those early days, nothing blatant, nothing overt.

My first friend in the neighborhood was a white woman named Barbara, who was born in Bermuda. Having lived in Bermuda, a country that is predominantly Black, she was comfortable with me and my family. She baked cookies for Wayne, who was five then, and our three-year-old, Sharon. She also offered to help babysit, invited us to use her phone while ours was being connected, and invited me to her church, St. Bartholomew's Episcopal Church. One Sunday morning, the children and I went along with Barbara. It was nothing like St. James Episcopal in Lafayette Square, the heart of the Black community. At St. James, the mostly bourgeois parishioners dressed to kill. If you were a struggling woman without much money, like I was then, you didn't feel a part of the congregation.

I worked some weekends, and after going a few Sundays with Barbara, the children and I missed a Sunday. That week I got a call from the priest, Father Jack Malpas, telling me that they had missed my family in church and asking if I planned to return. I did, and today, more than fifty years later, I remain a member. Over time, I became the "parish nurse," the person the other congregants called if someone got sick or had surgery. I'd go to their homes to help bathe them or take care of other needs. And even in my neighborhood, the children came to know me as the nurse whose house they'd run to if one of them fell and got hurt.

Baltimore City Hospital was a microcosm of the city at large. The majority of the hospital's clientele were Blacks and poor whites, mostly without health insurance. These patients sought care at the City Hospital, where they would receive care regardless of their ability to pay.

I worked in obstetrics and gynecology. Amidst the joy of welcoming newborns into the world, we cared for young women recovering from botched back-alley abortions who came in because infection had set in. We saw the women who, in future years, would not be able to carry a pregnancy because of the damage they suffered from those illegal abortions, the pregnant mothers on the verge of delivery who had not had medical care for the entire term of their pregnancy, the women admitted with preeclampsia, with low-birth-weight babies struggling to survive. We saw it all, women whose conditions were worsened by their poverty and lack of access to proper medical care. I learned a lot from working in the obstetrics department. I helped deliver babies, scrubbed in for C-section deliveries, and looked after low-birth-weight babies in the neonatal intensive care unit who were struggling to live.

But I grew tired of training new registered nurses and medical interns. Because Baltimore City Hospital was a teaching hospital, there was a rapid turnover of interns whom I had to teach less technical duties like drawing blood and the various tubes to use. Once the new arrivals were trained and understood the hospital's processes and procedures, I had to step back in the shadows. The role of senior licensed practical nurse, with the additional training responsibilities, had been assigned to me because I had trained in England. Though I provided most of the care to the patients, there were certain limitations on the extent of care I could provide. Only *registered* nurses could assess patients and give the full range of care. I needed to return to school to obtain the more advanced registered nurse degree.

•

After I left Baltimore City Hospital, I spent a brief three months at Church Home and Hospital, where I requested time off for my daughter's fourth birthday party. I put in the request some two to three weeks in advance, received approval, and sent out invitations. Two days before the party, my supervisor rescinded my time off, telling me she had given the day to another nurse, who happened to be white. That nurse had requested time off to attend her brother's college graduation. Our supervisor felt the brother's graduation was more important than my daughter's birthday. I was irate. What they were telling me was that I was not important, my daughter was not important. I took the day off as planned, and when I returned my supervisor gave me a three-day suspension. I handed in my resignation letter.

That week, I got a job at Bon Secours Hospital on the west side of Baltimore, a Catholic hospital founded in 1919 by the Sisters of Bon Secours, Sisters of Mercy, Sisters of the Humility of Mary. Bon Secours Hospital in the mid-1960s served a mostly white population, a distinctly different set of patients than those who sought care at Baltimore City Hospital. It served the nuns from the neighborhood—Notre Dame of Maryland University and the Institute of Notre Dame.

One day, while I was giving an older nun a bath, we struck up a conversation, which inevitably turned to the issue of race and why I had come to work at Bon Secours. The nun and I had more conversations around race, which led to my first speaking engagement.

"Do you mind coming to the College of Notre Dame to talk about this?" she asked. "They're having a forum on race and discrimination."

I declined her invitation because I had never spoken in public before. She asked again, and I decided to give it a try. I talked about my experience at Church Home and Hospital—my first face-to-face encounter with blatant racism—and what it meant to travel with my family in North Carolina. Around that time, some of the nurses—all licensed practical nurses (LPNs) like myself—complained of unfair treatment at Bon Secours Hospital. They felt they were not respected, and the registered nurses, who were mostly white, talked down to them, assigning them more menial tasks. After we formed an in-house group, I called a meeting and invited the hospital president to listen to the complaints. But at the meeting, I was the only one speaking—the other nurses were afraid of losing their jobs. I ended the meeting early. I learned a good lesson: don't stick your neck out unless you're really prepared to lose your job. The administration respected me, however, for organizing the meeting and inviting the president.

These days when I talk to nurses, one of the questions I ask is whether they have heard about Mary Grant Seacole, the Jamaican-born nurse and heroine of the Crimean War. More often than not, the response is no, and so I tell them how Seacole learned her nursing skills from her mother, who operated a boarding house for wounded soldiers. Seacole's mother taught her daughter traditional Jamaican medicine, which she combined with Western medicine to treat patients. Though Seacole, a mixed-race woman born to a Scottish soldier and a Black Jamaican woman, was free, she had few rights. Nevertheless, she gained a reputation as a skillful nurse.

Seacole traveled widely, and in 1851, she traveled to Panama to join her brother. She opened a hotel, and soon treated and saved her first cholera patient. Seacole became known for her work treating cholera. In 1854, ten years after her husband's death, Seacole inquired at the War Office in England if she could be sent as an army nurse to the Crimea, a place with limited medical facilities for wounded soldiers. The War Office turned down Seacole's request, but she funded her own trip and established the British Hotel near Balaclava to serve the needs of sick and convalescent officers. She also visited the battlefield, risking gunfire, to nurse the wounded. Seacole was known for diagnosing cholera and later become known as "Mother Seacole."[4] Despite Seacole's work, she's often forgotten, her reputation overshadowed by Florence Nightingale, another famous nurse, who is white.

I tell Seacole's story because I know how easy it is for Black people to be overlooked, how hard we have to work to make our voices and concerns heard, how much we have struggled and continue to struggle to overcome prejudices of all kinds. And I tell that story because it reminds me of Stella, a poor woman trapped by racial and economic circumstances in Baltimore, finally finding a job as a school bus driver and looking for a way to take care of her family and herself.

•

Throughout the 1960s, race was always present, in big and small ways. The biggest, of course, was Martin Luther King Jr.'s assassination on April 4, 1968. News of Dr. King's death in Tennessee, where he had gone to support striking sanitation workers, passed swiftly through Baltimore. Just a day earlier, King had given a speech in which he said he wasn't afraid of death. King's death unleashed pent-up despair in the neighborhoods to which Baltimore's Black population had been largely confined due to decades-old zoning laws and redlining. Two days after his death, the city lit up. Cautioned to stay home, we—my husband, my children, and I—watched the looting and burning on television. My children, Wayne and Sharon, were about seven and five years old, too young to understand what was happening. I had never experienced anything like this, and like everybody else I was scared, wondering if my adopted city would never get back to normal. For nine days, rioters burned homes and businesses. My favorite stores were looted, but not burned. By the time it was over, six people had died, more than 700 suffered injuries, and 5,500 were arrested. More than 1,000 businesses were robbed, vandalized, or destroyed by fire. Away from Baltimore, in nearby Washington, DC, thirteen people died and more than 900 businesses were damaged.[5]

King's death incited the riots, but other social and economic issues contributed to the unrest as well. In Baltimore, especially, discriminatory housing practices dating back to the early part of the century created a domino effect on the economies of urban communities that lingers to this day. In his book *Not in My Neighborhood*, Antero Pietila examines the bigotry and residential segregation in the form of restrictive covenants, redlining, and blockbusting. During the Depression era of the 1930s, the Federal Housing Administration (FHA) under President Franklin D. Roosevelt's administration created the Home Owners' Loan Corporation (HOLC), which purchased mortgages in default and sold them back to the original borrowers at lower interest rates and more generous financial terms. This effort was intended to stimulate home ownership and construction-related jobs. To make the loans and reduce risk, the FHA drew up real estate risk maps for cities across the United States that were intended to prevent lenders from future bad loans. The FHA included residents' race, ethnicity, religion, economic status, and homogeneity in its assessment of the neighborhoods in each city.

In Baltimore, portions of the city largely populated by African Americans and Jews were coded red, meaning people purchasing homes in these urban areas encountered significant difficulty in obtaining mortgages. Neighborhoods around these urban areas were coded yellow. The government recommended that mortgages could be issued in these areas only with caution and strict terms. Few neighborhoods received the green designation, meaning purchasers in those neighborhoods were able to acquire mortgages at less restrictive terms. Of course, these neighborhoods were predominantly white.

Unable to access conventional financing, African Americans could only purchase homes through speculators, otherwise known as blockbusters, who provided financing at predatory terms. Using various tactics, these speculators coerced white homeowners to sell their properties at discounted rates, which the speculators then resold to Black purchasers at a significant markup. This white flight changed the racial makeup of the urban city centers.

By 1967, these discriminatory housing policies had created segregated neighborhoods, diverting resources to the predominantly white suburban neighborhoods. Burdened by the loan terms, income disparities, and policies that destabilized neighborhoods and denied the opportunities to build wealth via homeownership, Black Baltimoreans suffered. By 1967, these issues had compounded, making Baltimore ripe for the riots that broke out in response to Dr. King's assassination. Studies show that redlined areas are twice as likely to experience persistent poverty and more than three times more likely to show persistent poverty for at least five census periods.[6] In the immediate aftermath of Dr. King's assassination, the focus was on rebuilding destroyed neighborhoods and containing the violence.

But for a number of people, the riots awakened them to what I had seen then as a nurse: Baltimore City's racial dynamic needed to change to ensure the city's Black residents and poor residents were not left behind.

- PART II

COMMUNITY ACTIVISM

CHAPTER 5

Becoming a Community Activist

Once a month between 1960 and 1990, the Caribbean American Inter-Cultural Organization (CAIO) met in Washington, DC, or the Silver Spring area of Maryland in church basements, a member's dental office, or a member's home. The group was a mix of Caribbean nationals who had migrated to the area, some as students at Howard University, where CAIO was founded in 1958 to support the university's students, and others who were working adults when they migrated. By 1968, when I joined CAIO, it had become a nonprofit organization dedicated to promoting cultural relations among people from the Caribbean, Africa, and America.

I first heard about CAIO when I was invited to its annual independence and awards gala—an elegant affair held in a hotel ballroom in Washington, DC. Bill and I went, relishing the opportunity to dress in our finest formal wear, to dine amongst well-known civic leaders and honor those in our community who were working to better our lives. During the evening, I met a number of individuals—including cofounders and board members Leo and Carmen Edwards (then Carmen Nelson). Leo, especially, helped shape the political person I would become.

After the gala, I joined CAIO and sat in countless meetings with my fellow Caribbean nationals listening to the group's leaders and members talking about local, national, and international issues of importance to us all. Leo was a graduate of Harvard and leader in the

Caribbean community. He had a presence about him, a way of commanding a room. Month after month, he stood before the group of sometimes twenty or thirty people, talking about Caribbean unity and imploring us to get involved in the local politics of our adopted neighborhoods. Leo often talked about the importance of Caribbean people serving on local boards and commissions and running for public office. "We have children in schools and we pay taxes," he often reminded us. "We say we are going to go back to our islands, and fifty years later we find ourselves still here. We need to get involved."

At the time, fifty years sounded so far away, but now after living in America for sixty years, I can say: Leo was so right.

Many immigrants from the Caribbean considered immigration—whether to America, Canada, or England—a temporary step. Like the generations before mine that went to work in Cuba, Panama, and Costa Rica, my generation expected to spend a few years abroad working and accumulating wealth before returning to our island homes to live out the rest of our days. But, as Leo pointed out, our dreams of returning home didn't always materialize. We had children and built lives. Instead of living like temporary residents in our adopted communities, he said, we should become citizens and participate fully in the electoral process that determined the fate of our families and the amount of resources local and state governments allocated to education, policing, health, and a range of other issues.

So I did. I joined the Maryland Nurses Association, the National Black Nurses Association, and the Association of Black Cardiologists as a nonphysician member. I also served on the Urban Cardiology Research Center Institutional Review Board (IRB), which helped review the efficacy of medications for hypertension. The IRB's president was Dr. Elijah Saunders, a renowned national specialist on hypertension and cardiologist at the University of Maryland; its director was Dr. Wayne Kong. Later on, I also served on Dr. Saunders's Hypertension Interest Group that met at the University of Maryland. Through a grant, the group visited homes along with members of the fire department. Firefighters checked smoke alarms while the team, headed by Dr. Lennox Graham, checked the residents' blood pressure and made treatment recommendations. I started a Discharge Planning Interest Group and Quality Assurance Interest Group for nurses. I became involved in the National Medical Association and attended their meetings in Washington, DC. I joined the Black Congress on Health, Law and Economics and the Congressional Black Caucus Health Braintrust. On Sunday mornings at St. Bartholomew's Church, I sat in on discussions on education, health care, and economic development in the adult group classes. St. Bartholomew's has a long history of active participation in the civil rights movement. Father Jack Malpas, who served as rector during the 1950s and 1960s, was particularly active in social justice issues. He had joined the students during the lunch counter sit-in at Read's Drug Store and marched with various groups of protesters. With that visible role in social justice issues, the adult group class discussions at that time spanned a wide range, from religion to education, business, health care, or whatever topic was prevalent in the news.

I joined these groups to make a difference, and because I was unfulfilled. I was going to work every day, coming home, cooking, and going back to school and getting degrees, but something in me wasn't quite right. I was yearning to do something more. I went to church and prayed, looking for an answer. I started attending the meetings at church, but it wasn't until much later when I got involved in politics and ran for office that the feeling fully went away.

Month after month, I attended meetings and listened in without asking any questions. Still a relatively new immigrant learning the ways of America, I didn't think I had anything to add. So I sat quietly soaking up everything, separating the liberal ideas from the conservative ones, and knowing even then that the speakers I most agreed with were the liberal Democrats and those I disagreed with most often were the more conservative Republicans. These conversations helped shape my decision as to which party I would support based on the issues the party cared about.

At one point during this period, I served on twenty boards and commissions. But my commitments had a cost. I encouraged Bill to join me, but he didn't feel he fit in. We were already moving in different directions, ultimately toward a separation and divorce. Without knowing it, I was setting the stones that would mark my steps forward, toward a future in politics.

•

Long after I thought I was finished having children, I became pregnant with my third child. My second child, Sharon, was the only baby Bill and I had planned, and six years later, pregnant with my third, I had lots of reasons to worry. Sharon almost didn't make it. She had inhaled the meconium—a baby's first stool—and was in stress in utero. She remained in the neonatal intensive care unit after I had been discharged, and Bill and I spent her first days watching her through glass, unable to hold her. But she was a fighter. Six years after worrying about whether Sharon would live, I was concerned my third child would suffer the same fate.

Warren was born on February 3, 1969, the same date as his father and older brother. When the nurses put him in my arms he was smiling—three hours old and already smiling. But the biggest surprise was his birth date. To have one child born on the same date as his father is unusual, but having two sons born eight years apart share the same birth date as their father was highly unusual. Besides, February 3 was also the anniversary of my first date with Bill. So our young family had a lot to celebrate every February.

Preparing for a third child meant pulling back on some of my work, both at the hospital and with community organizations. After giving birth, I suffered from postpartum depression. I was used to earning my own money and being very active in my community. Staying home as a housewife and mother offered a different challenge I had not faced before. One, I was accustomed to spending without asking my husband for money. Without my income during the three months of maternity leave, our budget became very tight, leaving little room for me to spend at will. Two, I am a social person, and I like being out. Being confined at home with the baby, especially a baby who cried most of the night and slept during the day, as well as having never-ending domestic chores, led to a bout of depression. I began to have periods of anxiety.

Even so, returning to work full time created another set of problems, including finding adequate childcare for the three-month-old and after-school care for my older children. Luckily, I found an elderly lady in my neighborhood who was willing to help. Not long after having my third child, I returned to school. I enrolled at Edmondson High School at night, taking refresher courses in math and English. After completing those courses, I went to the Community College of Baltimore County in Catonsville, where they were offering the General Educational Diploma (GED) exam. After I had earned my GED, I enrolled in Baltimore City Community College, a school I had driven by time and time again, always telling myself that one day I would go there too. I wasn't satisfied with being in America working as a licensed practical nurse and feeling inadequate because of the limitations in the work I could do with patients. I would close my eyes and envision that I was at Baltimore City Community College. And I was able to execute that dream. That's how I have lived my life. I envision myself in places long before getting there.

In my first year I took sociology and psychology, and after I completed all the electives, I took the College Board's College-Level Examination Program (CLEP), which allows students to demonstrate their mastery of introductory college-level material and earn college credit.

Despite promises that I would get in after I passed the CLEP, when the nursing program started, I was not accepted. I was disappointed but waited for another chance. About a month after the program had started, I learned from classmates in my anatomy and physiology classes that four students had dropped out of the program. Knowing that, I made an appointment with the dean of Baltimore City Community College.

"I have three children at home and no time to waste," I said.

My next step was talking to the director of the nursing program, Mrs. Trudy Hodgers, and the faculty member who had the opening in her class, Mrs. Francis Hicks, so they could determine if I would be permitted to take the class. After I convinced them I could handle the classwork, I received permission to register. Class started at 1 P.M. that very same day. That's when I realized I had no money for enrollment.

I had, however, stashed away $250 in an account at the credit union at Bon Secours Hospital. I had to think fast about how to get the money in time to finish the registration process before class. This was long before ATMs and debit cards became part of everyday life. I called the credit union and asked that the person in charge leave a check for $200 with the switchboard so I could pay the tuition and buy my books. I had to plead since it was against the credit union's rules to leave a check with the switchboard.

Another obstacle: I didn't have a car. I walked down the hall and looked up and down, hoping to find someone I knew. Then I saw a Jamaican man named Rev. Ivan Haye, a respiratory therapist student. I explained my predicament and asked for his help, and thankfully he was able to take me to the hospital to pick up the check, and I could get back in time for class. I registered and rushed over to the bookstore to buy the used books, and within an hour I was standing in the door of the classroom, smiling triumphantly at my friends in the class, Betty Lee and Martha Land, nurses I had worked with at Baltimore City Hospital who knew I was trying very hard to get in the program. Milda Lewis, who knew me through my mother in Jamaica, and Barbara, Betty's sister, were also in the class. They all clapped when I entered.

Since the program had started a month earlier, I had a lot of catching up to do. The students had already taken their first major exam.

I yelled out, "Who takes the best notes in the class?"

"I do," Betty yelled back.

I had to work hard to catch up. I asked for the names of the female students who had dropped out of the class, and after class I went to one student's house to purchase from her the required class uniform and cap. I promised to pay her for the clothes since I had no more money. She was much taller than my five foot seven inches and heavier than me. So I spent the night sewing a four-inch hem in the skirt and hand stitching the sides because the very next day I had clinical practice at Baltimore City Hospital.

That first evening of classes before I got home, I called my son, Wayne, who was then about nine years old, and asked him to give his sister a breakfast dinner—waffles or cereal—and feed his baby brother until I got there.

"Mom, I got it," Wayne said.

Returning to school was not good news to Bill, who raised holy hell when I got home. "How could you dare go back to school with three children and you're working full time? Have you lost your mind?"

He carried on so badly most of the evening that I developed a full-blown migraine headache, complete with blurred vision. That night I was also studying for a clinical exam scheduled for the following morning. With the headache, I couldn't read, and Betty had to talk me through what I needed to know. Somehow, I passed with a score of 84. Bill never came around to the idea of me pursuing further studies, and he stopped doing some of the things—like picking up groceries and making dinner—that he had been doing before. He made my life very uncomfortable while I was in school.

My work schedule added to our troubles. We had had a plan to cover childcare. Bill worked from 7 A.M. to 3 P.M. and I worked the afternoon shift from 3 P.M. to 11 P.M. While that schedule meant we only needed a babysitter for a brief period in the afternoon to cover our commutes, it also meant Bill had to bundle the children up late at night when he had to pick me up. Many nights, I could not leave immediately after my shift ended because a patient had died or had a cardiac arrest. On those nights, Bill became upset. He thought I could have come out earlier. He didn't understand the protocols of our shift changes and the requirements that ensured that oncoming staff had a full report of the patients and their respective needs.

I thought a second car would help ease the problems. In addition, it would reduce my commute. I bought a second car, a little 1973 red Vega, but Bill was less than thrilled. He did not want me to drive. He wanted to take me where I needed to go. But from Bill's perspective, the second car meant I was too independent. He was no longer in control of where I went and how I got there. But for me, there was no turning back. I kept the car and kept on with the classes and with my job.

When I bought the car, I had just learned to drive, and I still had to get a driver's license. Bill had tried teaching me to drive the stick shift car we owned, but our lessons were fraught with tension. Eventually, I took driving lessons, and when I didn't have enough money for that, a girlfriend taught me.

Despite Bill's misgivings about me returning to school, buying a car, and asserting my independence, two years later, when I walked the stage to accept my associate of arts degree in nursing, he was there with our children in the audience, cheering me on.

As a graduation treat, we rented an RV and took the children to Disney World. I was looking forward to relaxing, but even before we left Baltimore, problems emerged. The RV Bill rented wasn't ready, delaying our departure. Then he decided to take his wheelchair-bound mother along. Imagine the challenges of navigating an RV and a crowded theme park with a wheelchair. On the way back, the RV broke down, and an already-expensive trip became even more costly. We stayed in a hotel, spending the day negotiating with the RV rental company to pick up the extra costs and get us a replacement vehicle.

When we got back to Baltimore, I found out our financial situation was even more tenuous than I thought. Bill and I had an arrangement: he would handle the bills while I was in school. But he hadn't been paying all of them, putting us in a situation I hadn't expected to be in. For the first time, I found myself at a Consumer Credit Counseling center looking for a way to reduce our debt and make us solvent again.

But the new degree and passing the boards also brought something else: a new job in hospital administration at Lutheran Hospital of Maryland writing policies and procedures, setting up the criteria to audit quality of care, developing standards of care, and managing the hospital accreditation process through audits and corrective action so the institution would be prepared when the accreditors came. I was no longer directly involved in patient care but on the other end identifying problems and coming up with corrective actions by using all my nursing skills. These skills would prove essential in my political career.

•

With nursing school behind me, I returned to community activism, even stepping up my involvement. In the middle of 1977, I called the campaign office of Councilman Norman Reeves, who represented my district and who was running for reelection to the Baltimore City Council. Councilman Reeves had many of the same goals I had—to help the needy and less fortunate. I was drawn to his vision and wanted to help in whatever way I could to see him reelected. Evening after evening, I knocked on doors, encouraging my neighbors to reelect Councilman Reeves. Much later, after he became ill and died, his wife, Iris Reeves, took his seat, and I worked on her campaign as well.

And there were other campaigns I worked on in the late 1970s and early 1980s: Sandy Rosenberg and Jim Campbell for the House of Delegates; Tessa Hill for the Democratic State Central Committee; Rikki Spector for Council and Senate; Stuart Simms for State Attorney; Barbara Mikulski's campaign for the United States Congress and later again when she ran for the United States Senate; Maryland congressman Kweisi Mfume; Baltimore mayor Kurt Schmoke; and many others. One thing was common among all the campaigns I worked on: each candidate had the same goals and objectives as I had.

Like any campaign volunteer, I did everything from licking stamps to handling campaign mail, knocking on doors to contact prospective voters directly, distributing campaign literature, and engaging with voters at the polls. On occasion, when Tessa Hill could not make it to meetings, while I was chair for her State Central Committee Campaign, I spoke on her behalf and began to learn another side of politics to which I had not yet been exposed.

Along with volunteering for the campaigns of various politicians, I was also contributing in other ways to community health initiatives via the Black Women Consciousness Raising Association (BWCRA) in

Baltimore. When I joined around 1978, the organization was run by Dr. Louise Johnson. Dr. Johnson was also very much involved in the political work of the Black Caucus. I accompanied her to meetings, learning from each new interaction about issues of concern to Black communities, how to develop policies, and numerous aspects of community building. Between these organizations, I got a good education of the behind-the-scenes work of developing policies that benefit our communities. I later served as vice chair of BWCRA, and Dr. Elaine Simon, who was from Antigua and was also part of BWCRA's board, did a good job during that time to market the organization.

Among other initiatives, we developed programs to expose Black women from the local communities to policies and the work that goes into forming policies, and we held workshops on lover-to-lover relations, mother-daughter relations, stress management, and how women could learn to feel good about themselves. I, too, had a lot to learn about stress management and building relationships. Even as I was doing this work in the community, my marriage was failing.

Dr. Maxie T. Collier, a psychiatrist who later served as Baltimore City's first African American health commissioner from 1987 to 1990, was so impressed by our work that after giving a talk at one of our programs, he asked me to help him set up a similar group for men. I worked with him to get the group going. Dr. Collier also went on to produce a program on local radio addressing issues related to men and men's health with Richard Rowe, whom I had initially recruited for the board of the Black Mental Health Alliance for Education and Consultation.

At that time, I was also a member of the HUB Organization, which promoted Blacks doing business with Blacks via monthly networking meetings. The HUB Organization was started by Henry J. Parks Jr., who owned and operated Parks Sausage Co., famous for its catchy television commercials with the "More Parks Sausage, Mom, please" jingle. Later, Raymond Haysbert and Dorothy Brunson—owner and operator of the WEBB radio station in Baltimore and the first African American woman to own and operate a television station with her purchase of WGTW-TV Channel 48 in Philadelphia in 1986—served as presidents of the organization. I learned a lot about business from these giants and from other business leaders who were part of the organization. I later served on the board of HUB.

Dorothy was a mentor to many, including Catherine Pugh, who was later elected mayor of Baltimore. Because of Dorothy's keen business sense, she served as my first campaign treasurer for many years. Much later, when Dorothy was diagnosed with cancer, I would go to her home many times to help take care of her, just as, before she became seriously ill, she had brought me herbal teas if she knew I was sick. Dorothy would succumb to cancer, and the day when we heard she was near the end, Catherine and I joined Dorothy's family at her bedside in the hospital in downtown Baltimore. We remained at her bedside until she took her last breath. We hugged, screamed, and cried. I had lost a friend and a champion, and Catherine had lost her friend and mentor.

When I was increasing my involvement in those many organizations, I didn't have a strong sense of where it would lead me. I didn't yet know that I was headed toward running my own political campaign.

•

Perhaps the thing that began to bind my work in health care and my burgeoning political activity was a greater awareness of the history of Black people's lives in America and the long fight toward civil rights. Until 1976, I had not known about W. E. B. Du Bois' *The Souls of Black Folk* or the work he had done to address the declining health of African Americans.[1] I didn't know about Booker T. Washington's talk in September 1895 at the Cotton States and International Exposition in Atlanta, Georgia.[2] Neither of these men's work were part of the literature or material taught in any school I attended or course I had taken.

But in 1976, while still working on the administrative side at Lutheran Hospital, I attended a meeting of the National Medical Association in Washington, DC—the largest and oldest national organization representing African American physicians and their patients. Since

I was a member of the National Black Nurses Association, I was allowed to attend. I was excited about the possibilities such a meeting could offer. Presenters discussed disease and death among African Americans and ways to bridge the gap between Black and white health care outcomes. I was completely blown away by what I was hearing. This was the first time I had heard the term "bridging the gap," and together with the history of the work of Du Bois and Washington and many other African American leaders to address health care for African Americans, I was getting a real sense of the disparities in health care for Black Americans.

I left the meeting motivated to get more active and involved with the national and local chapters of the National Black Nurses Association. Because of my involvement in these organizations, I learned about the Congressional Black Caucus Health Braintrust led by Congressman Louis Stokes. When Stokes retired from Congress, Delegate Donna Christensen, the representative from the US Virgin Islands, took over the leadership of the Congressional Black Caucus Health Braintrust and continued to bring issues that were pertinent to Black communities to the forefront. As a medical doctor, she had a good command of the issues.

I read *The Souls of Black Folk*, took more classes on Black history, and started paying closer attention to these issues. Du Bois's 1903 autobiography shifted the way we look at race and racism via the concepts of the color line, the veil of race, and double-consciousness—always looking at oneself through the eyes of others. Du Bois, through his extraordinary analysis, also assessed the progress of the race, identified the obstacles standing in the way of that progress, and offered solutions on how the nation could continue to dismantle the systems that stood in the way of forward progress.

A few years later, in 1906, Du Bois published "The Health and Physique of the Negro American." The monograph was one of a series of research studies published under the auspices of Atlanta University, a historically Black institution. Using census reports, vital statistics, and insurance company records, Du Bois documented the poor health status of African Americans in comparison to white Americans. Du Bois argued that the differences between outcomes for Black people and white people was a result of social conditions and not inherent racial traits. "With improved sanitary conditions, improved education, and better economic opportunities the mortality of the race may and probably will steadily decrease until it becomes normal," Du Bois wrote.[3]

That same year, scholars, health activists, and health professionals gathered at the Eleventh Conference for the Study of Negro Problems to discuss Du Bois's findings. The group adopted several resolutions, including calling for the formation of local health leagues to provide information about preventive medicine. The group also called upon health organizations to implement programs specifically designed to address the health care needs of African Americans.[4]

Washington's 1895 speech, which is often referred to as the "Atlanta Compromise," marked the first time an African American was tapped to give remarks to a racially mixed audience in the South. Washington suggested that African Americans should not agitate for political and social equality. Instead, as a group, African Americans should work hard, earn respect, and acquire vocational training in order to participate in the economic development of the South. That approach, he believed, would earn African Americans the respect of white society, as well as the rights of full citizenship. In 1915, Washington, who by then had become the principal of Tuskegee Institute and president of the National Negro Business League, moved the league's health week program to Tuskegee to give it a national focus. Washington considered the national health week effort to be critical for the advancement of African Americans. "Without health . . . it will be impossible for us to have permanent success in business, in property getting, [and] in acquiring education. . . . Without health and long life all else fails."[5]

I was determined to increase my knowledge. I bought some books and borrowed others from the library. As I became more interested in health disparities, I joined the Congressional Black Caucus Health Braintrust. The group met regularly on Capitol Hill in Washington and brought a range of prominent speakers from across the country to speak on disparity issues. And I became actively involved in the Black Congress on Health, Law and Economics (BCHLE), driving down to Washington, DC, on a regular basis to attend meetings. These groups were filled with the brightest health professionals who were committed to addressing inequality wherever they saw it.

Attending these meetings in Washington, DC, and walking the halls of the US Capitol was exciting, and I committed to taking advantage of every opportunity to learn about the issues affecting our communities and understand how legislators introduced policy and built coalitions. During this time I met Congresswoman Shirley Chisholm, the first African American woman in Congress and the first woman and African American to seek the nomination for president of the United States from one of the two major political parties. I sat at her feet and learned from her. I also met Dorothy Height, who served as president of the National Council of Negro Women for forty years, and C. Delores Tucker, the convening founder and chair of the National Political Congress of Black Women. Meeting these women and attending workshops, I learned about not only health disparities but politics, the role strong Black women played, and how to run for office—lessons that would play a role when I launched my own campaign.

Even after I had won my seat, I continued to attend meetings of the state and national organizations. Some of the legislation I proposed came from issues the panelists and attendees discussed at these meetings. I understood how important it was for legislators and the administration to work on solutions at the local and state level for problems that we saw in communities across the entire United States. To return year after year and report on programs and initiatives that I had put in place to solve problems I had learned about at the Black Caucus meetings was deeply satisfying.

When I began to understand racial and health and health care disparities—the higher burden of illness, injury, disability, or mortality experienced by one group of people relative to another—everything that I had seen as a nurse at Baltimore City Hospital began to make sense. The cause was exactly as Du Bois had defined it in his 1906 monograph: "The present differences in mortality seem to be sufficiently explained by conditions of life."

Over the years, a complex set of factors and events had limited opportunities for Black people across the United States. In Baltimore, which had declined from its heyday as a major industrial city, the factors seemed more acute. I was beginning to better understand how each of these factors created barriers for low-income and Black and brown people to access quality health care and services, compared with white Americans and those who were wealthier. I was beginning to see how much addressing disparities in health and health care mattered and the great cost of health disparities. And disparities are responsible for more than premature death. In 2018 racial and ethnic health disparities cost the US economy $451 billion, a 41 percent increase from the previous estimate of $320 billion in 2014.[6]

Across the United States, the African American community has taken steps to address health inequities, such as creating hospitals, medical schools, and professional societies, particularly when segregation limited their access to health care. When Booker T. Washington moved the health week program to Tuskegee, African Americans embraced it. Over a fifteen-year period between 1915 and 1930, African Americans in thirty-two states participated in the health week activities, and in 1935, more than 2,000 communities provided reports of their National Negro Health Week activities. Organizers saw it as their goal to make the health week activities a year-round program and to ensure federal authorities were paying attention to the health disparities affecting African Americans.[7]

By 1930, the health week activities were being run by the United States Public Health Service (USPHS), a change the Tuskegee organizers saw as a positive step toward making African American health care a part of the national public health agenda. Within two years, the USPHS established the Office of Negro Health Work under the direction of Dr. Roscoe C. Brown, a Black dentist, marking the first time since the end of the Civil War that Black health care issues were institutionalized within a federal bureaucracy.[8] That office operated until 1950, and its closure reflected the idea that separate programs and facilities for African Americans represented the ideals of segregation.

Despite all that earlier work, in the second half of the twentieth century, African Americans were still fighting to bring attention to the disparities contributing to higher incidence of mortality among Black people in America. Paying attention to the history and current issues, I began to understand the ultimate goal: health equity, reducing and eliminating disparities in health and the factors that contribute to the differences in outcomes. Health equity means not only attending to the needs of people who are at the greatest risk of poor health but also achieving a high standard of health for all.

My knowledge expanded due to the work I did at Lutheran Hospital in the inner city. My bosses—John P. McDaniels, who later became president of MedStar Health; John Green, who went on to serve as deputy secretary of health for the state of Maryland in the Department of Health and Mental Hygiene (DHMH) and vice president of MedStar; and William Jews, who later served as the chief executive officer of CareFirst Inc.—allowed me to go to Annapolis to participate in Senator Larry Young's monthly breakfast on health issues. Each of these men played a role in my growth in health care, and the breakfast meetings gave me an opportunity to see what it was like working in Annapolis, to learn how health care impacted the people of Maryland, and to get to know the people at the table. Senator Young also created a Black health study group where we began to look deeply into some of the underlying causes of racial disparities in Maryland.

I still had a lot to learn. Then in the summer of 1980, I flew to Dallas, Texas, for the Black Congress on Health, Law and Economics meeting, where nearly 10,000 professionals from a range of disciplines—social workers, medical doctors, nurses, psychologists, psychiatrists, dentists, lawyers, and representatives from various business organizations—gathered to discuss strategies for bridging health care gaps between Blacks and whites. The keynote speaker was Dr. Patricia Harris, the first Black woman to be named Secretary of Health and Human Services under President Jimmy Carter.

I returned to Baltimore from the meeting in Dallas excited about starting my own Black health congress in Maryland. Two years later, I was the founder of the Maryland Black Congress on Health, Law, and Economics (MBCHLE), bringing together Black nurses, doctors, dentists, psychiatrists, psychologists, and social workers, as well as representatives from the HUB Organization, the Maryland Dental Society, the Monumental City Medical Society, and the Monumental City Bar Association. Ironically, the Monumental City Medical Society was chaired by Dr. Basil Morgan, a Jamaican ophthalmologist; Dr. Gladstone Davis, another Jamaican who also chaired the Maryland Dental Society; and Dr. Horace Lesley, a Jamaican who was a dentist and the first treasurer of MBCHLE. It was heartwarming to see other immigrants from Jamaica having a leadership role in key health care organizations serving Baltimore City and the state of Maryland.

In 1983, one of our first tasks was addressing the University of Maryland Medical System's efforts to move from a state-run hospital system to a privately run organization. Black employees are usually the last hired and the first fired; I was concerned that this would happen to the licensed practical nurses at the hospital, many of whom were Black. That was the first time I was angry enough to show up at the Black Caucus meeting at the Maryland House of Delegates in Annapolis. To my surprise, member after member got up and left the meeting, only to return a short time later. I felt they were disrespectful to the public who had come from across the state to have their voices heard and to participate in the democratic process. Not until I became a member of the House did I understand why the members drifted in and out of meetings. Their movement was not disrespectful. Rather they left during the proceedings to give their own testimony before various committees that were meeting at the same time.

Nothing came of this meeting, however. That was another lesson I learned: well-connected and powerful lobbyists can easily work to get bills passed or derail necessary proposed legislation before it has a chance to become law.

Dr. Morton Rapoport, then president of the University of Maryland Hospital, attended a MBCHLE meeting to explain the actions the hospital would take. He reassured us that he would try to preserve as many jobs as possible. I was happy to see that our efforts had a good outcome and that, as an organization, we were effective.

•

The following year, Dr. Maxie Collier, whom I had met through my work with BWCRA and who was then head of the Black Psychiatrists of America, brought a social worker from the VA Hospital, Fikre Workneh, to meet with me to talk about research findings and his concerns about the misdiagnosis of Black men with mental health issues. Based on published research, Workneh found that Black men were often given the most serious diagnosis even when their behavior and symptoms didn't warrant it. In response, we cofounded the Black Mental Health Alliance for Education and Consultation in 1984 to make referrals to doctors and host cultural competency workshops to take the stigma out of mental health. Workneh was the first president of the Black Mental Health Alliance, and I was the vice president. Again I convened a group comprising two members from each medical discipline: nurses, psychiatrists, psychologists, social workers, medical doctors, and business associates. We hosted conferences and held cultural competency workshops to educate both Black and white doctors on cultural issues that were likely to lead to the misdiagnosis of Black men. Dr. Patricia Newton, a renowned psychiatrist, taught the first class at Crownsville Hospital in Maryland's Anne Arundel County. The conference, which was well attended, began the process of educating Black and white mental health professionals about the importance of cultural competency. This work continues to this day, with more emphasis on the importance of mental health diagnosis and treatment in the Black community, as well as fighting to remove the stigma of mental illness.

Getting a grant to pursue our work wasn't easy. Just like the Black men whose culture was misunderstood, we ran into roadblocks trying to explain how culture can impact diagnosis and why our organization needed funding to pursue its mission. Within months after founding the Black Mental Health Alliance, several of our members—Dr. Doris Starks, Dr. Janet Stevenson, Dr. Maxie Collier, and a few others—met one evening to write a grant to help fund our work and pay staff.

The doctor in charge of disbursing the grant money was Jewish and from a different social and economic class than the groups we were representing. Four of us from the Black Mental Health Alliance met with the organization as part of the application process, and I saw immediately how the differences in social and economic class were reflected by even a simple grant application.

"Why do you come to get a grant?" the doctor asked us that day. "My community is Jewish, and we don't come asking for those grants."

"You come from a more affluent community," I said. "We need the grant."

I went on to explain how important our cultural competency workshops were. "If a Black man comes to your office," I said, "with long dreadlocks and dressed in red and green and black colors, sits down and tells you that Haile Selassie is his savior, talks about *The Children of Sisyphus*, and tells you that he smokes marijuana or ganja as part of his religious ritual, you would think that's the craziest Negro you ever met. Right?" I described the typical Rastafarian culture, and the Jamaican novel, *The Children of Sisyphus*, which probes Rastafarianism and life in the Dungle, the rubbish heap where poor people take up residence. Only by talking to the doctor about these factors and showing him how cultural context could influence a diagnosis were we able to get the grant. With that money we hired an executive director to run the organization and move it forward.

•

The grant application process reminded me of the long, deep struggles African American communities continued to face trying to bring attention to the factors that influenced disparities in health care and trying to give disadvantaged people access to quality health care.

Cultural differences was one. Two years after my experience fighting for a grant to properly set up the Black Mental Health Alliance, the US Department of Health and Human Services (HHS) released its comprehensive study of racial and ethnic minority health. The *Report of the Secretary's Task Force on Black and Minority Health*—released in 1985 under the leadership of former HHS secretary Margaret Heckler with research conducted by Dr. Thomas Malone—confirmed the stark reality we were trying to change: 60,000 Black people die needlessly each year because they don't have access to quality health care.[9] The Black Mental Health Alliance was trying to address that very issue as it pertained to mental health.

The Heckler Report, as it was called, found that while the health status of Americans had improved, a disparity in the burden of death and illness experienced by Black and brown Americans persisted when compared with the overall population. In spite of the growing depth of scientific knowledge and the capacity to diagnose, treat, and cure disease, many persons in African American, Hispanic, Native American, and Asian/Pacific Islander communities had not benefited from the science or the systems responsible for translating and using health sciences technology. The discrepancy was evident in the life expectancy rates. By 1983, the life expectancy rate for white Americans was 75.2 years but only 69.6 years for Black Americans—a life expectancy rate that white Americans had already achieved in the early 1950s. Researchers were seeing a lag of about 30 years. The study found a similar lag in infant mortality rates. In 1960, the infant mortality rate among African Americans was 44.3 infant deaths for every 1,000 live births, roughly twice the rate for white Americans, which was 22.9. By 1981, the rate among African Americans had declined to 20 infant deaths per 1,000 live births. Again that rate was twice that of white infants, 10.5, and similar to the white rate of 1960.

The Heckler Report identified six causes of death that accounted for more than 80 percent of the mortality observed among Black Americans and other minority groups compared to white Americans: cancer, cardiovascular disease and stroke, chemical dependency (measured by deaths due to cirrhosis), diabetes, homicide and accidents (unintentional injuries), and infant mortality. Other factors that affected the overall health needs but were not tied to a specific disease included minority needs in health education, health professionals, and health care services and financing. These latter factors were among those the Black Mental Health Alliance was attempting to influence through educational programs for doctors pertaining to mental health treatment for Black men. I knew the problem was bigger than mental health care for Black men. We couldn't tackle this issue by addressing Black mental health care alone. Still, we carried on, putting on conferences and education programs to address disparities in this area.

•

At the same time that my political activism was gaining steam and I was making inroads to address disparities in health care, my marriage was falling apart. I was trying to fix these big, national issues but could not fix my own personal issues. Outside of work and school, I was failing. For a long time I had known my marriage wasn't working. But I wasn't willing to say I had failed. I didn't want to fail at anything. In the first five years of our marriage, culture and other differences caused clashes on how we raised our children. Had it not been for my parents being in another country, I would have left the marriage in the very early years. I don't give up easily, though, so I decided to stay and work on my marriage. The more energy I put into my children, my community, school, and full-time work, the less time I had for taking care of my husband. Looking back, I can see some of the issues, including financial and money management concerns, that ended our marriage.

Nineteen years after our wedding, Bill left. We needed time apart, he said. I found out accidentally what "time apart" to Bill really meant when my youngest son, Warren, returned from a weekend with his father with the news that his father had set up home with another woman. In retrospect, I should have known because my youngest son had come to me time and time again to tell me that his father had a girlfriend.

"Mommy, Daddy's got another woman," Warren said. "And he doesn't talk to her like he talks to you."

"Go away," I'd say each time, refusing to acknowledge that he was right until the fateful weekend when he returned to tell me he stayed with his father and his new girlfriend.

I wasted no time and filed for divorce that Monday, and in 1980 we finalized our divorce. Nothing about divorce is easy. It is painful on both sides. Wayne, my eldest son, had just gone off to college, so I was left to raise two children alone. Each child took the breakup of our family differently. Wayne was worried about me. It was a hard situation for a young man going off to college and leaving home for the first time to worry about his mother. Sharon, a daddy's girl, rebelled, blaming me for her father's decision to leave. I had a rough time trying to keep her in school and focused. Three years after the divorce, Sharon dropped out of Morgan State University, eloped, and moved to Alaska with her husband. She was only nineteen. I was raging mad.

My mother was the wise one. "She has a husband now," Mama said. "It's no longer your problem. It's his."

As my marriage collapsed, so did everything around me. Within a week or two of Bill leaving, the hot water heater died. The refrigerator broke down. My car, a little red Vega, wouldn't start. The roof started leaking, allowing water to drip into the bathroom. With everything collapsing, I did too. Overwhelmed, I found myself on my knees, hugging the toilet bowl and bawling. In the midst of it, I heard a voice saying, "Shirley, you're the one who has been holding this family together all along. You're not a bad person to depend on." I looked around and saw no one. The voice was so clear, I was sure someone had spoken.

Sobbing still, I got up and made my way to my bedroom. On my bed was an unopened envelope from a dear friend, Bernice Branford Lewis, that had come in the mail that day. She knew of my problems with Bill and had sent me a poem, "Footprints in the Sand." I read it again and again, holding on to the words, "When you saw only one set of footprints, [i]t was then that I carried you."

I cried again, but I also moved to fix the problems. I called a co-worker, Dale Hinson, who had told me about someone who fixed her roof. She gave me the name and he came immediately. I called another friend, Betty Lee, who suggested I call the gas company to replace the water heater. She explained that I did not have to pay the full bill at once but could pay over time as the full cost was incorporated into my monthly utility bill and spread out over several months.

I still had the problem of the refrigerator and my car. I went to Levenson & Klein, a now defunct department store on Route 40 West, and introduced myself to the manager. I told him of my plight, and after asking where I worked, he promised to have a fridge delivered by 5:30 P.M. that day.

By then I had been taking the bus to and from work for a month. I remembered an acquaintance had told me about a Jamaican mechanic who lived in my neighborhood, one street away from me. That day, I walked over to his home and spoke with his wife. Later on that evening the mechanic came to my home and introduced himself as George Taylor. He looked at the car, replaced the battery and oil, and placed air in the tires. He also showed me how to do these things myself. It was an old car that leaked constantly, and I needed to be prepared for emergencies.

"How much do I owe you?" I asked.

"Nothing," he said, noting that he had heard about my divorce and my new state as a single mother.

He was also a minister, and he asked that we pray together. We prayed then. I was grateful that I had managed to take care of all these things so quickly and easily. To this day, Bishop Taylor and his family hold a special place in my heart.

•

In the midst of the divorce, I was still enrolled at the University of Maryland and was stressed on one hand by the divorce itself and on the other by the reports I had to turn in. On one long weekend, I took a trip to Jamaica to rejuvenate. I remember sitting underneath an almond tree and Papa standing nearby telling me one of the sayings he lived by: "A high-minded woman is good for the life of any man, and the one who doesn't know it does not deserve her."

Those words helped me then. Even today, I live by the words he told my siblings and me over the years. He didn't like lazy people and he often repeated Henry Wadsworth Longfellow's "the heights by great men reached and kept were not attained by sudden flight, but they while their companions slept, were toiling upward in the night" as a reminder of the value of hard work. He often said that if you know one way to do something and someone is showing you another way, be quiet and learn what the person is showing you because in the end you will know two ways to accomplish the same task. I used to repeat it to my children and grandchildren, and once I was in the car and told my grandson which way to drive. He drove the way he knew, turned to me, and said, "Remember what Great-granddad said. Now you know another way."

My father's other favorite sayings pertained to friendships and attitude. He always said one shouldn't lend money to friends or relatives but we should instead give the amount we can afford to lose. What he meant was that our friendship or bond wouldn't be broken by the expectation of loans being repaid.

After I returned from Jamaica, I continued to think about what Papa said, blending it with what I gleaned from counseling sessions. Just before my marriage ended, I had started counseling to deal with the ongoing stresses that were causing my daily migraines. Dr. Frank Beckles, who was referred to me by my church sister, Inez Haynie Dodson, taught me to practice the biofeedback method and along with counseling helped me gain more control over my body's normal involuntary functions. By using the power of the mind and becoming aware of what was going on inside my body, I could gain more insight into my health. Whenever I started feeling stressed, I knew to get away from it and practice a relaxation technique. It really helped me, and later I started teaching seminars on stress management.

"When you were married," Dr. Beckles said, "you had a husband who bought you gifts at Christmas, for birthdays, and for other important events. Now treat yourself. Always save some money for things you want."

That's the best advice I had heard. The first year, I put a diamond ring on layaway, taking a year to pay it off. For the next big holiday, I put a mink coat on layaway. I went on that way, saving for years to treat myself to something big—a trip to England, another house, the Mercedes Benz I dreamt of each morning when I sat on the bus. On the bus, I also drew pictures of the Mercedes Benz that I dreamt of owning. Each of these physical purchases restored some sense of accomplishment in a life that felt like it was falling apart. I carried on. My educational and professional investments added up, too, leading me to take a bigger step toward a life in politics.

CHAPTER 6

Early Response

Implementing Care

The Moselle and Rhine rivers wind through villages that I had only ever imagined from the fairy tales I read as a child. Set amidst the hills were ancient castles, vineyards, and harbors of breathtaking beauty. For two weeks in 1985, I visited the Netherlands, Germany, Belgium, and Holland, tasting Gouda cheese in the city where it's made; buying a small diamond in Antwerp, the diamond city; wandering through Bruges, a city famous for its lace; with the prince; touring the Ahr Valley; visiting the Van Gogh Museum and the Red Light District in Holland, as well as the Rembrandt Museum; dressing up for medieval dances in Frankfurt; sitting in the Grand Plaza in Belgium tasting as much of the local wines and beer I could stomach. The ship, the MS *Amicitia*, took us up the Moselle and Rhine rivers, stopping at various ports where I shopped, buying way more than I needed and worrying about how I would take all my purchases home. I had won the two-week FAM trip thanks to Beatrice Reed—a real estate broker, former president of the Caribbean American InterCultural Organization (CAIO), and grandmother of comedian Dave Chappelle—who had put my name in a drawing.

But my mind kept turning back to Baltimore, my home now for twenty-five years. Sitting on deck, I started jotting down notes about my community in Hunting Ridge and the problems—big and small—I had seen there and across Baltimore. I made notes about the issues I encountered in my role as a board member of Planned Parenthood and House of Ruth Maryland and about running the Maryland Black Congress on Health, Law, and Economics. I had ideas to address some of these problems, and even in Europe, far from the source of my concerns, the ideas kept coming. On that trip—thirteen years after I met Stella in the hospital room at Bon Secours Hospital and thought about what needed to be done to change the inadequate laws governing health care—I made the momentous decision to run for office. It was time, I thought, to do a little more.

The decision wasn't made lightly. A year earlier I had given it some thought, even meeting with Congressman Parren Mitchell's campaign manager, Terry Taylor, for advice. When Taylor told me that I would need at a minimum $10,000 to run a campaign, I was taken aback.

"If I had $10,000, I would have invested it in the stock market," I said.

But I didn't have that kind of money. Where would I, a nurse living paycheck to paycheck, get that kind of money? I had set the thought aside, but here I was a year later, jotting down ideas and fully ready to start campaigning.

Two weeks after I got back home, I invited some friends over so I could pitch them the idea. Nearly fifteen of us—friends from church and colleagues from work—filled my living room, spreading out in the dining room chairs and on pillows on the floor. Amidst the Jamaican patties, cheese and crackers, and drinks I set out for them, I placed an easel with a flip chart. On it, I had written my goals and objectives. I talked about the things I had done, including my association and involvement with Planned Parenthood, the National Black Nurses Association, the Maryland Nurses Association, CAIO, and various boards.

But what I really wanted to hear from them was whether I was the kind of person they thought could represent them in Annapolis. Each friend and coworker said yes, boosting my confidence and confirming my dream. That evening, I raised $1,500. My largest contribution came from Ruth Goodwin and John and Judy Hayes, both members of St. Bartholomew's Church, which has a rich history of activism. They continued to support me throughout my efforts to run for office. It wasn't until years later when Ruth Goodwin died that I learned she had served as treasurer of the state board of the League of Women Voters and that during the 1950s and 1960s she and her husband, William Goodwin Jr., were active in the civil rights movement. I finally understood why she had such a vested interest in my success.

With the first campaign contributions, I opened a Friends of Shirley Nathan-Pulliam bank account and started my first run for office, in 1986. Before I could fully begin, I had one other task: telling Kweisi Mfume that I could no longer volunteer on his campaign for the US House of Representatives. Telling him was complicated. I was running on a ticket with delegates Sandy Rosenberg, James "Jim" Campbell, and Wendell Phillips. Then-delegate Phillips was running against Kweisi for the same seat in Congress. Understandably, Kweisi was disappointed.

We dubbed ourselves the "CPR team"—Campbell, Pulliam, and Rosenberg—because we were fighting to resuscitate the community by concentrating on key issues that were most important to all of us: education, health care, economic development, criminal justice reform, and the environment. Our goal was to infuse new ideas into the community and bring it back to life. To reach our constituents, we mapped out the areas and streets where we would each campaign. I concentrated on the Black communities where I was well known, the very communities where I had worked for years on the campaigns of many elected officials.

In the summer of 1985, following a ceremony honoring Michael Manley, former prime minister of Jamaica, he learned I was running for public office and offered to campaign alongside me. But at the time, Mr. Manley had a strong relationship with Fidel Castro.

"If I come to campaign with you, you may lose the race," he said. "Because of my relationship with Cuba, they think of me as a communist."

Although he was unable to support my campaign, I was grateful for the offer and overjoyed that he would even think of wanting to help. I was struck again by Mr. Manley's warmth and charisma, and how easy it felt to talk with him.

Because of my work with the various Caribbean organizations in Maryland and Washington, DC, I had the opportunity to meet with the former prime minister on many other occasions at the home of Leo and Carmen Edwards and in the company of Ambassador Curtis Ward—including one event in the summer of 1988, when Mr. Manley came to promote his book, *History of the West Indies Cricket*. And in June 1993, Mr. Manley came to Washington, DC, accompanied by Dr. Peter Phillips, who was then a rising politician in the People's National Party, for a ceremony honoring the former prime minister and launching the Jamaica National Development Foundation. My best friend, Millicent McLeod, Ambassador Richard Bernal and his wife Margaret, and I attended the ceremony at the Organization of American States.

Election morning—November 4, 1986—my son, Wayne, and I got out early. Wayne was my driver for the day, taking me from one polling station to another where I made myself known, shaking hands and talking with constituents, pressing brochures into the hands of voters who had not yet decided which candidates to support. In the late evening, after the polls had closed and we were on our way to the house where the other delegates on my ticket were gathered, I heard the results. Campbell and Rosenberg won their races, but I lost my race by a very narrow margin. I cried in the car, then went in and celebrated their wins.

The lessons I learned then about running and managing a campaign influenced all my future campaigns. Even now, they stay with me. One particular lesson is that every polling place where you are on the ballot should be covered by your campaign volunteers and those who have your interests at heart.

•

Fresh off that loss, I returned to Hopkins to finish coursework toward my master's degree in administrative science business management. I had started that program in 1983 because I wanted to start my own business. To build a successful business, I needed to understand how to write a business plan, prepare a marketing plan, and look at finances. I wanted to study something practical.

I had stopped my studies temporarily to run for office, but with the campaign behind me, I put everything into completing the degree and launching the business. Besides, I stood to lose credits if I did not return to the graduate program. My biggest problem with completing the degree was once again money. I had none, having spent what little I had on the campaign. But I was determined to find a way.

With the new term about to begin, I went to the Johns Hopkins campus with a check made out for $500 and a promise to pay off the rest of the tuition if the university allowed me to take the remaining twelve credits. They did—something that wouldn't happen today. But with that promise, I finished those twelve credits. For my final paper, I created a business plan for a health care company providing health services in homes and consulting on health care issues. As I was working on the business plan, I started seeing patients little by little while still working at Liberty Medical Center.

On a cold day in May 1988, I walked across the stage with Papa and my stepmother, Mae, looking on to see my achievement. They were in Baltimore visiting from Jamaica for Wayne and Judith's wedding, which had taken place a day earlier, and they came with me to the university that morning. My father was proud of what I had achieved, but he also thought that I was accumulating degrees to prove myself to him, harking back to my childhood learning disabilities.

"Shirley, you can stop proving me wrong," Papa said that day.

My father was indeed correct. I wanted to prove myself to him. But it had taken me some time to get to this moment where I could so easily let go of any lingering resentment toward him. Several years earlier I had gone to Jamaica with Bill and the children, and when I greeted my father I didn't embrace him. I didn't feel any warmth toward him and kept him at a distance. Back in Baltimore after the trip, I wanted to tell my father exactly how I felt. Throughout my childhood, my father had spent willingly for educational activities for my siblings, who didn't struggle with learning as I did. He paid for my siblings to take the Common Entrance Exam that determined whether children in the sixth grade proceeded to a traditional high school or went on to a vocational secondary school. And when my siblings passed the exam, he willingly paid for them to attend prestigious high schools.

I sat down and wrote a ten-page letter on the pages of a ruled yellow legal pad. I wrote about the things he could have done differently to help me learn, how much it hurt when he put me down in front of my siblings and pitted them against me by asking them to recite multiplication tables at the dining table when he knew I couldn't. All the resentment poured out of me.

I folded the thick wad of paper, put it in an envelope, and headed to the post office.

"Five dollars and fifty-five cents," the mail clerk said.

But I had only a dollar. I couldn't mail it. I took the letter back home. Time passed and the envelope moved from one part of the house to another, until it was permanently lost or I threw it out. But the act of putting my feelings in writing changed something within me, and the next time I saw my father, I could hug him without hesitation. I could look at him without resentment and see him as a self-assured man who had worked hard to raise five children, a man who owned his own property and owed no one money.

Here I was in Baltimore, working hard not just to prove Papa wrong. Not only was I stubborn, but I was also motivated by the idea that if I worked hard, I could achieve what I set my mind to. I always remember what my father said of completing tasks and attitude: "Prove yourself. If you can't get a job done right, don't do it at all." I was probably fourteen when he first said that, after I ironed the collar of his shirt and did not get it straight, even though I thought I had done a good job. From that time I always remembered to do my best in everything.

•

That same year—1988—Providence Hospital merged with Lutheran Hospital and became Liberty Medical Center. I stayed on with the merged company as a quality assurance coordinator. I worked pretty hard on quality assurance concerns to save the hospital thousands of dollars in fines from accrediting bodies by going through reams and reams of memos and converting them to policies and procedures. By writing out the step-by-step procedures for staff in various departments across the hospital and establishing criteria for auditing the charts and the related hospital units, I helped establish patient standards of care. But one thing had changed. Before the hospitals merged, while at Lutheran Hospital I worked with Dr. Mary Etta Mills, the nurse health consultant, to write the standards of care and set up audit criteria. Dr. Mills was also responsible for getting me to earn bachelor's and master's degrees.

"For all the things you do, writing standards, you cannot continue to have an associate's degree," she said. "You have to move on."

All along, I had been thinking that I was working and taking care of my children. But Dr. Mills's advice was the best anyone could give me. Then and later on she was there for me.

Under the merged company, I was assigned to a supervisor with even fewer qualifications than I had—something that was baffling, given my experience and education. My supervisor, a white woman, had an associate's degree, and I had a master's degree. I felt my skills, experience, and education weren't appreciated.

Around that time, I was scheduled to attend a conference in Washington, DC. My nursing administrator, who was very knowledgeable about hospital accreditation, supported and approved of me attending the conference. Yet my new supervisor, with no good reason, wanted to prevent me from attending. I was upset. Trying to understand, I went to speak to the then president of the hospital, William Jews. But he couldn't offer any specific information, except to say that the hospital had to make administrative changes. I went to the conference anyway.

Back at work the following day, my supervisor said, "I have to write you up."

"You don't," I said. "Here's my resignation letter."

Surprisingly, I was not nervous. I was confident that I had made the right decision. After thirteen years in that position, I felt that I deserved to be treated with more respect.

During my last month at Liberty Medical, I went to the state health department to file paperwork to formalize the personal health care business, which I named Nathan's Networks and which I ran for nearly thirty years. I assigned nurses and nurse's aides to help patients with their personal care and activities of daily living, anything from bathing patients to moderate cleaning to getting them to and from doctor's appointments. I didn't need much to get the business started, just a desk, two chairs, a filing cabinet, and a computer. I found an office to rent and set out to enroll clients.

•

One morning, about a week after I returned to Baltimore from a vacation in Jamaica, my stepsister, Faye, called to say Mama had a stroke. Mama's stroke occurred the day after I had left Jamaica, but at Mama's insistence Faye and my stepfather waited a week to let me know what had happened. Mama had told her and other family members to not bother me with the news because she knew I would have to turn around and come right back. But a week later, when they realized Mom was not improving, they called. I got myself together and flew back as soon as I could.

When I got to Mama's home, I found my mother extremely depressed. Mama was a big lady, but I climbed into bed with her and rocked her. Tears streamed down my face. Mom was completely paralyzed on the right side of her body, and she couldn't take care of herself. Back then, the Jamaican hospitals sent stroke patients like my mother home; there was no hospitalization, no treatment, and no physical therapy, none of the treatments that were standard in America at that time. Part of my role as daughter and nurse and caretaker was convincing Mama that God had not put a curse on her and that the stroke that paralyzed her body was a result of her not following the doctor's orders, failing to take her prescribed blood pressure medicine and follow her dietary restrictions. Before I left Baltimore, I had packed a book of illustrations on how high blood pressure can cause a stroke, from the formation of a clot until the actual stroke occurs. I came prepared because I knew Mama would say that God was punishing her by giving her a stroke.

I stayed in Jamaica for two weeks. I contacted her physician, ensured she got her blood drawn, and set up a contract with a physical therapist and a nurse to take care of her. A few months later, Mama decided to come to America to receive better health care. I bought a hospital bed, a commode, and a wheelchair. Her husband, John, accompanied her on the trip. Outside the airport terminal, Mama, who was in great spirits, stopped the wheelchair. She eased out of the chair and stood to her full height of approximately five feet nine inches.

"Beauty, sit down," my stepfather said. He was worried that she might fall.

Mama hushed him. "Wait a minute." She took a deep breath and with some flamboyance, said, "I'm in America," with great emphasis on the word "America."

Even with a stroke, nothing was going to stop her from doing what she wanted to do. Her spirit and her determination to survive were strong, but what Mom could do was limited. I bathed her and cooked meals before I went to work. My children, adults by then, sometimes helped with dinner. But taking care of her and getting her to and from physical therapy was rough. And if it was rough for me, a nurse with extensive knowledge of medical care, what of the families with no such knowledge? What must it be like for the sick confined to their homes? I thought about the homes I visited in my new role running Nathan's Networks. Some homes in the summer were so hot I could barely breathe, and in the winter months they were extremely cold.

I thought about opening an adult medical day care so patients like my mother could socialize and improve their quality of life. Typically adult day care centers give a bit of relief to caregivers while ensuring that the patient is cared for in a safe environment. Some adult day care centers focus primarily on social interaction, while others provide medical care or specialized care for patients with memory loss or cognitive impairment. I talked to two girlfriends who opened adult day care businesses. But I held off until 2000. It wasn't the right time for me to jump into another business venture because of my legislative responsibility as an elected official.

But I could not get the idea out of my mind. I had a deep desire to open an adult day care, largely because of the physical conditions of the homes of some of my clients and what I went through with my own mother. When I opened that business, Mama's memory was embedded in my actions. A photo of her in her wheelchair was on the brochure, and her name was included in every aspect of the business. I didn't want to forget why I opened the day care and who I was serving— the elderly, the disabled, and those with strokes like my mother. During that time I was also working part time in a rehabilitation hospital, then called Montebello Rehab Hospital. I worked in the head trauma unit, avoiding the stroke unit. It's hard as a medical-surgical nurse, wanting to see immediate results and knowing that recovery from strokes is slow.

•

That fall when Mama visited me in Baltimore, I hosted a second celebration of life party for her and my special friends. I had been holding these parties at either my home, church, or business since 1984 as a way to tell my closest friends and family why each were special in my life. Sometimes I had the women arrive first for conversations around women and our needs. The men joined us later for drinks. At the heart of each of these parties was my talking to each person individually to say why he or she was special in my life. Sometimes I recited Maya Angelou's "Phenomenal Woman":

Pretty women wonder where my secret lies.
I'm not cute or built to suit a fashion model's size
But when I start to tell them,
They think I'm telling lies.

At the party for Mama, Halloween decorations were still on tables arranged in the parish hall at St. Bartholomew's. We'd told Mama she was going to a concert, and she got all dressed up for that occasion. Her hair was swept up in a bun, and she looked regal. My sons wheeled her into the hall, and as soon as she realized I had planned the celebration for her, she began to cry. She cried the entire evening, in part because she was overcome and partly because the stroke had affected her ability to control her tears. As I walked around the room thanking my friends and telling them why they were each important to me, she cried some more.

Within four years, she passed away.

"I know you're busy doing fifty things," Mom often said. "If you get a call that I died, take your time. Don't break your neck to come. I'll be waiting for you."

As we talked on the phone about my plans for Christmas and her birthday, I remembered her words. She was upset that I couldn't come home that year, 1992. I wanted to be in Jamaica, but there were too many things to get done in that last month of the year and in the last few weeks leading up to the Caribbean inaugural ball I had planned alongside a Republican, St. George Crosse, in honor of President Bill Clinton's January 1993 inauguration.

On a cold January morning, my stepsister Faye called to tell me Mama had died in her sleep. Mama's birthday was December 11, and she died on January 10. I couldn't help but think of the belief that most people die within a month of their date of birth. Not being there for Mama's Christmas is one of my greatest regrets. But we sent her off beautifully, burying her on my granddaughter Brianna's sixth birthday in a plot in the very community cemetery Mama had adopted and raised money to keep clean for many years.

At the funeral, I spoke about my mother coming to visit me in Kingston when I was a little girl. One day, she came for a parent teachers association meeting wearing a black-and-white dress with a peplum, and matching black and white shoes. My mother was tall and stately, and stood out to the children around me. For most of my childhood, my mother was a buyer and saleswoman for a popular department store in Montego Bay and was always well dressed.

"Who's that lady with you?" the children asked.

"Oh, that's my mother," I said.

"Shirley, you can lie." Nobody believed she was my mother.

Sometimes, as a child, I didn't believe either that she was my mother, thinking instead that my Aunt Clara, my mother's sister, was my mother, because of our close resemblance and because my birth certificate stated that she was present at my birth.

Everyone knew Mama as "Miss Beauty." I wanted Mama to be remembered not only for her outward beauty but that she was, as Bette Midler sang, "the wind beneath my wings," a woman I always looked up to and admired. And I didn't want to forget that the experiences I had taking care of her in the latter stages of her life mirrored the experiences of so many people in my community who had access to care but nevertheless received inadequate care and services.

•

Four years after Mama's death, I went through the same thing again, this time with my father. My sister Harlene called to say Papa had a stroke. He was still living in Kingston, and I rushed to Jamaica to help take care of him. A few days in, I began to sense Papa's discomfort with me bathing him and taking care of his personal needs. He was a very proud man.

One day as I was trying to feed him, he resisted, clamping his mouth shut. No matter how much I coaxed him, he wouldn't open his mouth.

"Papa," I said. "Are you trying to tell me something? Are you trying to tell me that you want to die?"

Because of the stroke, he was aphasic and unable to speak properly. But he opened his mouth and said clearly, "Yes, yes."

With tears in my eyes I walked away from his bed. A few days later, I returned to Baltimore. But within a day after flying back home, I got word that Papa had died, and I returned to Jamaica to bury another parent.

With all that experience caring for family members with strokes, it is easy to understand why operating an adult medical day care was so important to me. I understood what families experienced, and I wanted to, in some small way, ease their burdens.

Though both of my parents were in Jamaica when they had their strokes, cardiovascular disease was a significant problem that I saw in the African American population. I wanted to address that problem and the underlying disparities. So in 2001, I proposed legislation that shifted the focus of the existing State Advisory Council on High Blood Pressure and Related Cardiovascular Risk Factors. The advisory council was renamed as the State Advisory Council on Reducing Death and Suffering from Heart Disease and Stroke. The legislation required the council to develop and promote educational programs on heart disease and stroke prevention. It also required the council to recommend that the Department of Health establish guidelines for the effective management of heart disease and stroke, which included high blood pressure and other risk factors, and required the council to evaluate the heart disease and stroke prevention, education, and treatment programs.

CHAPTER 7

Later Response

The Path to Public Service

One Monday morning in 1992, a personal care aide from Nathan's Networks whom I had assigned to care for a blind patient called after finishing up a visit. On that morning's visit, the aide found the patient, Mary—an elderly woman in her nineties—still wearing the diaper the aide had put on the patient on her last visit the previous Friday. Mary had been wearing the same diaper for three days and nobody in her household had changed her. Besides Mary's general discomfort, such neglect presented a number of potential concerns, not least of which were Mary's skin breaking down and leading to bedsores, or her developing a urinary tract infection. If Mary's diaper had not been changed in three days, had she received her necessary medications? Had she been fed? What other aspects of her care had been neglected? I went to the house to follow up.

Three generations lived in the house—Mary, along with her daughter who was about seventy years old, and Mary's great-grandchildren. Mary's daughter answered the door. One of the girls, very young at the time, clung to the woman's skirt. Mary's daughter also needed a nurse. She was obese and had a number of obvious health issues, and she was in no condition to be taking care of her mother. I learned that the children's parents were incarcerated, and the elderly grandmother was, for the time being, the children's caretaker.

We climbed a set of stairs to the second floor. The stairs shook under the woman's weight, and I didn't think they were strong enough to hold both of us. I waited until she cleared the staircase before following her. Upstairs, I found Mary in a dark and smelly bedroom. There was no window, and the only air circulating in the room came from a single fan perched on a chair.

"Good morning, Miss Mary. How are you today?" I asked.

"Don't my daughter know that I am hungry?" was Mary's only response.

The little girl was present still, except this time she held on to me instead of her grandmother. "Nurse, nurse," she called.

When I looked down at her, she pointed to the fan. I saw what had scared her. Trapped on the blades of the fan was a dead mouse, going round and round, spreading the scent of death in the room.

"Why didn't you put your mother in a nursing home?" I asked the daughter.

"I promised my mother I'd never put her in a home," the daughter said.

But I couldn't leave Mary there. I called 911 and requested that an ambulance come to transport Mary to a hospital. Weeks later Mary died in the hospital, but I rested easier knowing she was no longer hungry, didn't die in filth, and received the care she needed.

Mary's case reinforced one of the biggest holes I encountered in the health care delivery system across my job in nursing, running an adult personal care and health care company, and serving as a social services commissioner for the Baltimore City Department of Social Services. Access to health care was one thing. Access to *quality* health care was another thing altogether. Patients like Mary had access to health care via Medicaid, but they did not necessarily have access to quality care and services. Health disparities were—and still are—high among the mostly elderly populations Nathan's Networks served. What I saw reinforced what I had known from my first meeting with Stella: we ought to do a better job of providing adequate care for all communities and demographic groups across the state. Elderly patients were especially vulnerable.

Around the same time I encountered Mary, Maryland's Board of Public Works, which oversees the administration of the state's significant expenditures, was attempting to cut services for the elderly and vulnerable patients. The proposed cuts would eliminate the personal care program for the elderly—the very program Mary had relied on for help with her basic needs. Any such cuts would be devastating to a significant number of the patients Nathan's Networks served. I rallied fellow nurses to support my lobbying effort against the cuts. We didn't go alone. We took a group of elderly residents from the Baltimore area—some in wheelchairs, some mobile and intellectually disabled—to Annapolis to show who we were fighting for. The hearing before the Board of Public Works is held in the State House in the governor's reception room. That particular meeting was televised and, for the first time, I saw myself on television standing before the state's governor, comptroller, and treasurer testifying passionately to save a program I believed in.

I wanted the members of that body to put themselves in the shoes of the elderly who were dependent on the program slated to lose its funding. I asked them to consider one question: If you were sick in bed and didn't have the money to pay for help and had no one to help you, what would happen to you? I had come forearmed. At the time, I knew that the wife of the state comptroller, Louis Goldstein, was sick. So I asked him, a working man and a wealthy man, "If you didn't have the money to pay someone to bathe your wife and turn her, how would she survive?" I asked the treasurer, who was also ill, the same question. Both knew exactly what my question meant. It struck their very core.

When the proposal to cut the services came up for the vote, both the treasurer and comptroller voted against it. Their vote meant the state maintained the program and the essential service for the state's senior residents. The governor was the sole member of that body who voted to cut the services. Our efforts had paid off.

At the end of the process I was certain of two things: I knew how to lobby, and I was ready again to run for office.

Every ten years or so, following the decennial census, Maryland's governor determines the boundaries of the legislative districts for electing the members of the Maryland General Assembly. Following precedent, after the 1990 census was complete, Governor William Donald Schaefer formed the Governor's Redistricting Advisory Committee (GRAC) to develop a redistricting plan. The GRAC made a series of changes, including creating a new minority district along the Liberty Road corridor in western Baltimore City and southwestern Baltimore County. This new legislative district—District Ten—covered my neighborhood. As a new district, no incumbent representatives would run for office there. Here was a chance for me to run again for the House of Delegates. Besides, having worked the polls each year at the neighborhood polling location, I was well known in the community. This new district gave me a great chance to win.

I jumped into the race, assembling a team of volunteers and staff, and getting on the campaign trail to reintroduce myself to the community and raise funds. Twenty-one candidates were vying for the seat, and I wanted to make sure the voters knew about my long-running involvement in the community, as well as my service on the boards of various organizations that impacted their lives. I ran on a ticket with Senator Delores G. Kelley and delegates Emmett Burns and Joan Parker. This time, on election night we were all together, watching television for the results. As the numbers came in, we were ahead. We would win our respective races and take our place in the Maryland General Assembly. I would become the first Jamaican and Caribbean person elected into the Maryland General Assembly.

In the days following my win, with everything still a blur, then delegate Kelley took me to the Maryland State House in Annapolis, marking the first time that I entered the State House through the garage. As she showed me where I would park, the enormity of what I had accomplished began to sink in. I, a Jamaican woman, who had migrated to the United States, had won an election to represent my Baltimore community in the Maryland General Assembly. And I would have a designated parking space, marked with my name on the wall.

Before me stood the vast Maryland State House, the country's oldest state capitol in continuous legislative use. Today it is the only state house to have once been designated the nation's capitol. Presidents Thomas Jefferson and George Washington served in that capitol. The Continental Congress met in its Old Senate Chamber from November 26, 1783, to August 13, 1784—during which time George Washington resigned his commission as commander-in-chief of the Continental Army, and the Treaty of Paris was ratified, marking the official end of the Revolutionary War.

Again I was overwhelmed by the magnitude of what I had accomplished. Seeing the vastness of the building and thinking of the importance of Annapolis and the work that delegates and staff conducted there was overwhelming. I was excited and apprehensive, and at the back of my mind a little question cropped up over and over. Can I do this?

Then I remembered: *Can't* is never in my vocabulary.

That day I handled some of the smaller details that would define my life as a Maryland delegate and member of the Maryland General Assembly. I selected the hotel where I would stay during the legislative session. The Maryland General Assembly meets for ninety calendar days each year beginning the second Wednesday in January and continuing through early April. This meant I had to move temporarily to Annapolis for each session. I completed the paperwork and signed the required contracts, then shopped for suits and dresses more fitting for my new role.

In the last week of November, the Maryland General Assembly legislative class of 1994 embarked on a ten-day bus tour to learn about Maryland's diverse communities and the range of issues that would come before us. We visited every corner of the state, journeying from urban cities to rural farm towns, learning about the pretty and not-so-pretty parts of the state and the overall machinery that makes our state run—the sewer system, soil conservation efforts, botany, waste disposal from ships docked in the waters off the Eastern shore. We observed crabbers. We learned how oysters are harvested. We learned about the invasive phragmite weed—a tall perennial grass found in wetlands—and how to control it. We visited Poplar Island, a manmade island in the middle of the Chesapeake Bay that the Maryland Port Administration and the US Army Corps of Engineers began rebuilding in 1998 with dredged materials. The island had been close to disappearing because of the forces of the wind, waves, and current when the engineers intervened and found a way to restore it and maintain a crucial wildlife habitat. We slept in bunk beds like teenagers at camp, sitting up into the night telling stories.

At the end of our trip I understood why the former Speaker of the House delegate Casper Taylor said of the legislature, "Every four years in the legislature is equivalent to a PhD." I had so much to learn. If I was going to make decisions, I had to ensure I had the right information and tools to make good decisions. Legislating, it seemed, was a little bit like tackling problems as a nurse. First you identify a problem, then you assess and plan how to solve it. Once you have a plan of action, you implement care. Finally, you follow up and evaluate the outcome. Everything I learned about nursing became part of my political career.

•

Wednesday, January 11, 1995, the first day of the legislative session, was a cold winter day. I had come southeast from Baltimore to Annapolis the previous day and settled into the hotel that would serve as my home base during the legislative session. That morning, I took my time getting ready, alternating between trying to settle my nerves, tamping down my excitement, and reminding myself why I had fought to take on this role and what I hoped to accomplish. Always at the back of my mind was how far I had come—from a young girl struggling to read to an immigrant and nurse to an elected legislator. Sharon and Wayne and Sharon's husband and daughters were on their way to Annapolis. My granddaughters, Brianna and Nicole, were then seven and five years old, and I was proud to have them witness this moment and to believe that they, too, could achieve what I had achieved—and even more.

We gathered in the State House, which was already brimming with members of the print and broadcast media, federal legislators who represented Maryland in the US House of Representatives and the US Senate, Maryland county executives, and mayors of cities across the state. Family and friends of the delegates were spread out across the room, some sitting in the balcony and some standing along the back wall of the chamber. My children stood in the back, and my younger granddaughter, Nicole, sat on my lap.

We celebrated but not long after the festivities wound down, the real work began. I had to interview and hire staff and deal with other administrative tasks of setting up and running an office. Now that I was in Annapolis, the center of Maryland politics, my roles and my life had expanded.

Mother. Registered nurse. Business owner. Community activist. Politician. I filled all those roles simultaneously and quickly had to learn how to juggle the demands of each role and handle multiple tasks at once. By the time I won my first election, my children were older— adults living independent lives who didn't need me daily. But I had a business that I needed to maintain. Running Nathan's Networks meant I had to make quarterly home visits to the hundred or so patients we served at the time. That was the registered nurse's job, and as the owner of the business I had long filled that role. Aides handled the other daily patient care duties. Now that I was a delegate, I had to make changes to how the business operated. To keep the business going, I hired a registered nurse to handle the tasks that I would otherwise have done. Other administrative tasks, like meeting payroll, I handled on the weekends when I went home. Sometimes I saw patients on the weekends. But I always made time for Sunday service at St. Bartholomew's Episcopal Church.

Fresh in Annapolis, I was itching to take on something big, to tackle the health, racial, and economic disparities that had plagued my health services career. But the first two bills I sponsored were not the deeply impactful bills I had long imagined. When I was first nominated to serve on the Social Services Commission in 1992, I was also serving on the Democratic Central Committee, which I had been on since 1990. But I was told I could not serve as a commissioner *and* on the Democratic Central Committee simultaneously. The law surprised me, since my work on the Central Committee would not have impeded my role as a commissioner. And there was no underlying conflict, since none of the two roles was a salaried position. In my first year, I sponsored and won approval of a bill to change that law.

The second proved to be more problematic. Delegate Campbell, with whom I had campaigned in 1986 for the Forty-Second District race, asked me to put in a bond bill to support the Girl Scouts of Central Maryland's efforts to purchase new headquarters. Almost immediately, Senator Kelley informed me that freshmen don't sponsor bond bills because they never get passed. She suggested that I pass the bill to a more seasoned delegate. As a freshman, I had not yet learned the unwritten rules; concerned that I had breached protocol, I asked Delegates Campbell and Rosenberg if either would take on the bill and see it through the House. But both refused to take it. It's your district so you should put it in, they both said. And both wanted me to get the experience of sponsoring bills.

I was worried about how I would get out of this bind. While riding the elevator, I saw Delegate Howard (Pete) Rawlings, who was then chair of the Appropriations Committee and responsible for bond bills. When I told him of my plight, he was more encouraging than I expected. "Put your bill in," he said.

I did as he said, but while my bill passed in the House, the companion bill failed in the Senate. Even with that loss, I learned a valuable lesson: a key part of legislating is building relationships with people.

•

Night after night, I sat up, poring through the bills, reading as much as I could to keep up. Sometimes I stayed up as late as 3 A.M., stopping only to catch a few hours of sleep before I got back to it again. Because of my dyslexia I am a slow reader, and I wanted to make sure I understood the nuances of the bills the committees on which I served were discussing, and all the other bills that would come to the floor for a vote. I wanted to make sure I was doing right by the people who voted for me and others across the state who depended on legislators and the administration to make decisions that would likely impact their health, finances, environment, or education.

But trying to read through bills that were sometimes hundreds of pages long was exhausting work, and difficult for a reader like me. The sheer volume of bills made it a daunting task. It's not unheard of for delegates to introduce hundreds of bills in a ninety-day session. Between 2013 and 2015, senators in the Maryland Senate introduced an average of 1,045 bills and 1,461 in the House. With the session lasting only ninety days, reading through all those bills in such a short time was difficult.

I took courses on speed reading and tried different ways of learning to read faster and be as prepared as possible for each day's meetings. Little did I know that my colleagues were not doing the same thing each night. They were not staying up, like I was, into the wee hours reading every line of the proposed bills. Instead, they read the fiscal note, which summarizes the corresponding bill and the projected cost to Maryland. With the thousands of bills introduced in each legislative session, it is important to know the price tag of each bill, the resources available to carry out the proposed initiative, and the potential revenue to the state. How the fiscal note is prepared can also impact a bill's chance of getting approval.

Reading the fiscal note instead of reading through every line of the bills saved me and got me on course to think through amendments that I thought would improve the proposals and lead to better results for Marylanders.

- PART III

KEY LEGISLATIVE INITIATIVES

Health Disparities

CHAPTER 8

Treating Cancers, One Bill at a Time

In the months leading up to the November 1994 presidential election, I got word that my best girlfriend, Harriet Bais Branch, had breast cancer. Harriet sometimes tutored me, and we spent many days studying together. Harriet was diagnosed with an aggressive form of cancer and underwent chemotherapy, radiation, and a mastectomy. I was with Harriet at her home the day she learned the treatments were no longer working. When I walked in, she was sitting in the basement of the split-level home. She had no expression, simply a blank look on her face. She looked sad and miserable. When I asked her what happened, she said, "They said they can't do anything more."

I screamed and bawled. "I will cry for you," I said because she wasn't crying at all.

Memories of Stella came rushing back. Here was another woman I had helped nurture through a cancer diagnosis on the brink of death. Unlike Stella, Harriet had health insurance and her cancer was caught early, but the aggressive nature of Harriet's cancer affected her outcome. Less than a month later, around 3 A.M. I got the call from Harriet's husband that she was near the end. I drove to her home as quickly as I could, held her hand, talked to her, and closed her eyes when she passed. Reliving all that Stella had endured was difficult.

Nearly twenty-six years after meeting Stella I was in a position to address breast cancer diagnosis and treatment in uninsured and underinsured women. When I met Stella in 1972, breast cancer was the leading cause of death from cancer for women in the United States. At that time, it was often diagnosed because of clinical signs and symptoms. The medical community had come a long way in diagnosing and treating breast cancer—from surgical biopsy in the operating room to image-guided, fine-needle aspiration or core biopsy in the radiology department and the routine use of mammograms to screen for changes in breast tissue.

Despite the progress in the intervening twenty-six-year period in the diagnosis and treatment of cancers and concentrated efforts to catch cancers early, a mammography screening program for low-income underinsured and uninsured women age forty years and over had expired. In the nearly four years that the program—conducted by Maryland's Health Services Cost Review Commission (HSCRC)—was in place, it had detected an estimated 500 cases of breast cancer. Yet it was allowed to expire at the end of June 1997 with no comprehensive replacement program in place for the thousands of underinsured and uninsured women who relied on it to get the mammograms they needed but could not otherwise afford. At that point, a federally funded program providing coverage to women over age fifty was still in place.

That year alone, 3,866 women in Maryland were diagnosed with breast cancer and 823 Maryland women died of breast cancer. Breast cancer was the second leading cause of cancer deaths among women after lung cancer. While white women had a higher incidence of breast cancer than Black women, Black women experienced higher breast cancer mortality rates than white women. Maryland women had the seventh highest breast cancer mortality rate in the United States.

I immediately thought of Stella, whose breast tumor grew unchecked because she didn't have the health insurance or the money to pay out of pocket and get the appropriate care. The HSCRC program would have benefited her had it been available in 1972. Without such a program, what would happen to women who had relied on it for care? I decided to honor Stella by proposing a bill that would make mammograms widely available to low-income Maryland women on a permanent basis. I recognized the need to not only continue the HSCRC program but also expand the existing federally funded Centers for Disease Control and Prevention's National Breast and Cervical Cancer Early Detection Program. I worked closely with the University of Maryland School of Medicine and the Greenebaum Cancer Center on the legislation, with significant help from Claudia Baquet, MD, and Dr. Priscilla Chatman, Esquire.

House Bill 766, as I envisioned it, would require the Department of Health (then known as the Department of Health and Mental Hygiene) to establish a breast cancer program to provide screening mammograms and clinical breast examinations to specified low-income women aged forty to forty-nine years at least biennially and provide annual screenings for women aged fifty years and older. The bill would require the program to diagnose and treat individuals in need. The bill would open the program to any Maryland woman aged forty years or older with a family income at or below 250 percent of the federal poverty level and who did not have access to health insurance coverage that covered mammograms and clinical breast exams.[1]

A chill had settled upon Annapolis that January of 1998 when the new session started. The session began with President Bill Clinton's scandal swirling around us and the very real possibility of impeachment proceedings. There was a buzz in the air, uncertainty over where the scandal would lead and how, if at all, the scandal and possible impeachment would affect Democrats across the country. In Annapolis, some thirty miles from the center of the scandal in Washington, DC, we put our heads down and went to work.

At the top of my agenda was the proposal to, at a minimum, restore the state program that made mammograms widely available to low-income Maryland women over age forty. For several years, the state had conducted a vigorous public campaign urging women to get their yearly mammograms. Given what was widely known about the effectiveness of early detection of cancers, I thought we had a good chance of getting HB 766 and the companion bill that Senate Republican member Jean Roesser sponsored in the Senate to the respective floor for debate and passage. I felt confident the bill would pass easily.

Yet the chairman of the Environmental Matters Committee blocked the proposed legislation. Since each General Assembly session meets for ninety days, I had a limited window to get the legislation to the floor and passed. Time and time again, I asked the chairman if he would bring the bill up for vote. But each time he objected to the breadth of the low-income women the legislation as written would serve.

"You need to bring it down to 150 percent of the federal poverty level," he told me one day.

"No, it needs to stay at 250 percent," I said. That threshold was also the standard set by the Centers for Disease Control and Prevention, and I didn't want Maryland's legislation to set a lower standard.

The 1997 federal poverty guidelines ranged from $7,890 for a single-person household to $26,930 for a family of eight. By the chairman's calculation, the income range under the bill would be $11,835 for a single person to $40,395 for a family of eight. From experience, I knew that basic medical services were often a hardship for a single person earning $19,725—250 percent of the federal poverty level. I knew the bill needed to cover a wider range of women who would otherwise be denied access to a service they needed and would not otherwise be able to afford.

I feared we would get to the end of the legislative session without the bill coming up for a vote. I pulled out all the stops to get the bill to the floor, arranging for women's groups to call the State House to encourage support for the bill. Day after day, the women's groups lobbied the chairman, yet he would not budge.

As we neared the end of the Assembly's session, I saw him in the hallway with his head down. He looked especially sad, and I asked one of my colleagues if something was wrong with the chairman. I learned his wife had discovered a lump in her breast. Later, I approached the chairman and asked him directly what was wrong. He confirmed what I had heard.

My nursing instinct kicked in. I put my arms around him and said, "Don't worry. Eighty percent of those lumps are benign." I emphasized to him that it was important that he be there at her bedside, holding her hand.

He thanked me for comforting him.

Three days later, I was sitting at my desk on the floor of the House, and he was sitting diagonally from me. There were a number of people around us, so I called him from my desk phone.

"How did things go with your wife?" I asked.

"It's benign," he said. "Thank God it's benign."

"Great," I said. "I told you not to worry."

Later that afternoon, when we got to our committee hearing, he asked if I had the votes to bring the bill up for a vote. Having gone through the cancer scare with his wife, he had a change of heart and was ready to move forward with providing coverage for a greater part of the population of poor women.

"Yes, I have the votes," I said. "I've had the votes all along."

I had already lobbied everyone on the committee for their support by reminding the men that they had wives, sisters, and mothers who have breasts and could face the same predicament of the women the legislation would cover. I did not have to push as hard to get the support of the female members of the House and Senate. None of the delegates wanted to say no to a bill like that and return home to their female relatives knowing that they stood in the way of diagnostic mammograms for women.

The legislation headed to the floor and passed unanimously, then was signed into law by the governor in May 1998. It provided $2.6 million annually for screening, diagnosis, and treatment of breast cancer in low-income women. The day after the signing we took pictures at the University of Maryland School of Medicine with the head of the Greenebaum Cancer Center, Dr. Claudia Baquet, Dr. Priscilla Chatman, and Councilwoman Beatrice "Bea" Gaddy, who had been previously diagnosed with breast cancer and died not long after.

Councilwoman Gaddy's death hit me hard. Gaddy, a Black woman, was an activist for the hungry and homeless. Every year, she hosted a large Thanksgiving dinner to feed hundreds of people in Baltimore. One of her dreams was to create a breast cancer center for low-income women in the inner city. But she died before we were able to accomplish this. Gaddy's activism had led to her being elected to the Baltimore City Council. But until she was elected to the council in 1999, she—like many others for whom she advocated—didn't have health insurance. Once she had health care coverage, Bea underwent chemotherapy treatments, and the cancer went into remission. But the cancer recurred in 2001, and in October of that year, she died. Once again, lack of access to health care resulted in late detection and likely cost Bea her life.

But in that moment after the bill passed, we had something to celebrate. The months of nagging had paid off, and I felt relief and a sense of pride that I had been able to secure breast cancer screening services for other women like Stella. But I was also disturbed that what it took to get the bill to the floor was not empathy or concern for the underserved, underinsured, and uninsured women but a medical scare that had threatened my colleague's own family. Was it likely that the only way to address disparities was by reaching my colleagues on a personal level?

Indeed, it was. Time and time again, I used that tactic when testifying in support of a bill. Since the Maryland legislature meets for ninety days in the first part of the year, many delegates continue to work in their respective fields, including education, medicine, and emergency medical service. To get a bill through, from time to time I had to say, "You're an EMS, a fireman. Walk with me in the situation where you could get infected."

Much later, I relied on that same tactic to get a chemotherapy parity bill through. I put a senator's wife's name on the bill, calling it the Kathleen Matthias Chemotherapy Bill. The bill addressed the differing costs of chemotherapy given to patients in a hospital setting versus those obtaining it on an outpatient basis. Chemotherapy charges for a patient in the hospital would be paid through the patient's medical plan, but when given outside the hospital setting, the cost of the drug was paid through the patient's prescription plan. The latter was more expensive. In some cases, patients were spending so much money trying to stay alive that they lost their homes and filed for bankruptcy protection. The bill created parity so the costs would be the same regardless of how the patient obtained the medication.[2]

•

Early in my tenure as a delegate, I began to understand invisibility in a way I never understood it before. I quickly started putting in bills to address some of the racial disparities in health care that I had encountered throughout my career as a registered nurse and as the owner of Nathan's Networks.[3] I testified about significant issues—infant mortality, HIV/AIDS, hepatitis C, and cardiovascular disease—all from the lens of race and the impact of these health issues on the Black community. But the people whose causes I championed remained invisible. I was simply not heard. I was dealing with a room full of predominantly white men from different parts of the state, most with a small percentage of Black residents. They weren't interested in or swayed by the statistics I was sharing on the morbidity and mortality of Black people across the state. I began to think that all my efforts were in vain.

The sense of invisibility was most clear to me at the time I was trying to push an oral cancer bill forward. At the time, African American men had the highest oral cancer rate in Maryland. In 1997, 562 Marylanders were diagnosed with oral cancer and 174 Maryland residents died from it. In that same year, the age-adjusted oral cancer mortality rate in Maryland was 3.0 in every 100,000 people, higher than the national oral cancer mortality rate of 2.5 per every 100,000 persons. Maryland was at that time seventh among the states and the District of Columbia in oral cancer mortality. For that same period, Black people were diagnosed with and died from oral cancer at a higher rate than white persons. In 1997, 11.4 African Americans out of every 100,000 persons were diagnosed with oral cancer versus 9.5 white persons. And for that same year, the mortality rate among African Americans was 4.1 out of every 100,000 persons, versus 2.8 for white persons. In addition, white Marylanders were diagnosed with oral cancer at an early stage in higher proportions than Black Marylanders—41.3 percent versus 31.8 percent.[4]

Armed with statistics and studies, I pressed my fellow delegates to pass the bill to address this high rate of oral cancers among Black men. Yet the bill that I put in was ignored. At the time, I was working with the University of Maryland School of Dentistry to get funding to treat the many homeless men who turned up with oral cancer. The cancer rate among that group of men was particularly high, with drug addiction, alcoholism, and poor nutrition exacerbating oral cancer disease. I worked closely with the dental school on the program to examine and treat this group of men.

Another delegate, Leon Billings, an outspoken white man representing Montgomery County, pulled me aside. "Nobody cares about Black people. Call it something else. Say it is for the low-income or underserved populations."

When I first proposed the bill, I wanted to name it the African American Male Oral Cancer Initiative to address the unique needs of Baltimore and the group of men in the city more likely to be diagnosed with the disease. But I also understood that getting the legislation passed meant I needed to broaden the language to make sure it covered underserved populations rather than specifically point to the race of a specific demographic group.

I was grateful for the feedback, but I wasn't surprised. None of my approaches had worked. But if we were only speaking about the poor and underserved, how would we address the racial inequities in health and minimize the adverse impacts of systemic racism? How would we develop policies that ensure Maryland's health care system provides access to high-quality care for all? The 1985 *Heckler Report* had already addressed the persistent health disparities that affected Black and brown Americans. Yet here we were just twelve years after the *Heckler Report* was published, ignoring race as a factor in legislation surrounding oral cancer care.

Indeed, cancer was one of the six causes of excess deaths among African Americans, the Heckler Report identified. Tobacco, dietary/nutritional factors, occupation, and ethanol were the major risk factors that accounted for 72 percent of all cancer deaths between 1979 and

1981, the time period covered by the *Heckler Report*. Tobacco was then the greatest risk factor for cancer for African Americans. Among Black men, tobacco-related cancers accounted for nearly 45 percent of new cancer cases and 37 percent of new deaths. Among Black women, tobacco-related cancers accounted for 25 percent of new cases and 20 percent of new deaths.[5]

Another significant finding from the *Heckler Report* was the differences in survival rate based on the cancer site. For 1976 to 1981, the five-year relative all-site survival rate was 50 percent for white persons and 38 percent for Black Americans. Of the twenty-five primary cancer sites for which survival data were available, Black Americans had better five-year relative survival than white persons for only three sites: ovary, brain, and multiple myeloma. Black patients had better survival rates than white patients for ovarian cancer for all stages combined and also within each stage category. When breast cancer was considered, the survival rate for Black patients was 63 percent and 75 percent for white patients. Researchers attributed the discrepancy to the large number of Black patients whose cancer affected the lymph nodes or whose cancer had spread beyond the primary site. Black patients also showed a lower survival rate for colon and bladder cancers.

Among Hispanic patients, the overall age-adjusted cancer incidence rates were lower than for Black Americans or white Americans. For Hispanic patients, the cancers that occurred more frequently affected the stomach, prostate, esophagus, pancreas, and cervix. Stomach cancer incidence in Hispanic patients was twice that of white patients.

Researchers concluded that social or environmental factors rather than inherent genetic or biologic differences accounted for the differences in cancer outcomes between white and Black patients, which meant we had an opportunity to address these factors with policy changes related to screening and detection, treatment, rehabilitation, and education for specific at-risk groups. When researchers adjusted data to account for the stage at diagnosis in cancer patient survival studies, survival differences between Black patients and white patients decreased. When adjustments for socioeconomic status were factored in, the disparities between the two groups were further reduced. The *Heckler Report* also noted several factors that may contribute to poor cancer survival in Black patients: lower socioeconomic status, later stage at diagnosis, delay in detection and treatment, treatment differences and biologic factors such as immune competence and response, histologic patterns of tumors, and nutritional status.

Given all the data we had, why were legislators and the administration ignoring the very real factors a significant portion of the population faced?

•

Later in 1997, the four largest cigarette manufacturers in the United States agreed to settle yearslong litigation that the state attorneys general of forty-six states, five US territories, and the District of Columbia had brought regarding the ways the companies advertised, marketed, and promoted cigarettes. As a signatory to the agreement, Maryland was slated to receive more than $4 billion over a twenty-five-year period. On the heels of that settlement, then governor Parris Glendening announced a ten-year plan for the use of the funds and created three task forces to develop recommendations, including the Governor's Task Force to Conquer Cancer in Maryland. The task force published a report in December 1999 outlining the guidelines under which money from the fund would be allocated. Reducing "disparities in cancer mortality, survival, and quality of life among minorities and persons living in rural and underserved areas of the State" was one of the key goals. And that goal was at the heart of the work I wanted to do as a legislator.

Once the Maryland General Assembly's 2000 session got underway, we began to deliberate on how best to allocate the funds. We established the Cigarette Restitution Fund (CRF),[6] as well as the process and requirements for distributing money from the fund. The CRF program's key goal was to implement strategies to reduce the burden of tobacco-related disease in Maryland. Key target areas were tobacco-use prevention and cessation and cancer prevention, early detection, and treatment. Through the CRF program, administered by the Prevention and Health Promotion Administration within the Department of Health and Mental Hygiene, Maryland created tobacco-use prevention and cessation programs; cancer prevention, education, and screening programs; cancer research programs; and a statewide network of cancer and tobacco local community health coalitions.

Following the release of the Report of the Governor's Task Force to Conquer Cancer in Maryland in June 1999, I decided to reintroduce the stalled legislation aimed at reducing oral cancer mortality among underserved populations. The Task Force's report underscored what I had been trying for years to get my colleagues to see: oral and pharyngeal cancer is twice as common in African American males than it is in white males. Largely preventable, the five-year survival rate of oral cancer is 52 percent when it is detected early.

Armed with the newly released report, I sponsored another bill concerning oral cancer. The bill required the Secretary of Health and Mental Hygiene to establish an oral health program that would develop a targeted program to prevent and detect oral cancer in high-risk underserved populations. Another mandate was the development and implementation of programs to train health care providers to screen and refer patients with oral cancers and to promote smoking cessation programs.

•

I wasn't done addressing breast cancer. Fighting for funding for breast cancer screening and diagnosis was only one part of the equation. The quality of the care mattered as much as having access did. In the case of Bonnie, an immigrant from Antigua, the care she received after a mastectomy nearly cost her life.

As Bonnie sat watching television one day, a news item about a free health screening caught her attention. At the time, Bonnie was waiting for her visa application for permanent residency to be finalized. She was without health insurance and did not want to miss the opportunity to catch up on some of the health screenings she could not otherwise afford. She went to the facility, where the medical team performed a series of diagnostic exams, including a chest x-ray. The x-ray showed a shadow, which sometimes indicates a serious underlying problem, and sometimes nothing at all. Bonnie was concerned, and she went to a hospital for further exams. There, the doctors diagnosed breast cancer and a treatment plan that included a mastectomy. But because Bonnie had no health insurance, the hospital where she was first seen did not want to proceed with the surgery. I stepped in, making calls to the hospital and another nearby facility to find a doctor willing to perform the mastectomy. I found Dr. Miles Harrison, a breast specialist, who agreed to treat Bonnie if the hospital where Bonnie was first seen refused to proceed with her operation. Fortunately, after receiving numerous calls from me, the original hospital where Bonnie was first seen agreed to perform the procedure.

The medical team instructed Bonnie not to eat on the morning of the mastectomy but failed to tell her not to take the insulin that she regularly took to manage diabetes. Prior to surgery, having gone without food for so long, Bonnie started to go into hypoglycemic shock, which delayed the start time of her procedure. Later that day, after she recovered, the surgeon proceeded with the mastectomy. Those days, mastectomies were considered outpatient procedures, with the patient sent home after a short recovery period. But at 5 P.M., when the ambulatory center was scheduled to close, Bonnie had not completely awakened from the anesthesia. The team, anxious to leave for the day, woke her up, put her in a wheelchair, and called her family to come get her. But Bonnie was in no condition to go home. She was in extreme pain, and her family members who had come to get her were so concerned about her condition that they called me for help.

Once again, my nursing instinct kicked in. "Take her to the emergency room," I told them. "Don't leave the hospital with her."

At the time, I was washing my car in my driveway, but I jumped in the car—wet jeans and all—and sped toward the hospital's emergency room. Bonnie was still sitting in the wheelchair, doubled over in pain. None of the staff members had done anything to help as yet. I stepped in as if I worked there, wheeled Bonnie to an empty bed in the emergency room, put her in it, and told the staff to get her some pain medicine. She was then seen by a doctor and medication ordered, and she was later discharged in the wee hours of the morning.

I left the hospital late that night sure of one thing: a mastectomy should not be a drive-thru procedure. No woman should be forced to go home immediately after such a major operation, especially if she does not have a support system in place to handle her care.

Still disturbed by the state in which the hospital discharged Bonnie and the inadequate instructions given to her family, I returned to the hospital to make a complaint. The nurse I spoke to that day—an RN with both a Bachelor of Science and a Master of Administrative Science degree—said she had had a mastectomy and didn't need all those instructions.

I was even more annoyed. "How could you, an educated registered nurse, compare yourself to the average person coming in, who doesn't have your training and doesn't know what to do? You cannot compare yourself. You have the same degrees that I have, and I know that all patients, regardless of their background, need to be given proper discharge planning instructions."

Something had to be done about patient education in circumstances like these.

After a couple of days, Bonnie continued to have issues. At home, the bags connected to the surgical drainage postsurgery were hung too high, so the fluid was draining back into her body, further contributing to her discomfort, fever, and pain. Her family again called me. When I heard Bonnie had a fever, I told them to take her back to the emergency room. That second trip, she received antibiotics and more pain medicine before being discharged again.

Bonnie's second trip to the hospital underscored the need for more supportive care for mastectomy patients, including discharge planning. In 2009, eleven years after winning the battle to get breast cancer screening, diagnosis, and treatment covered for poor women, I set about writing a second breast cancer–related bill. HB 41 and the bipartisan companion bill in the Senate would require certain insurers, nonprofit health service plans, and health maintenance organizations to provide inpatient hospitalization coverage for up to forty-eight hours following a mastectomy that is performed for the treatment of breast cancer, and to provide coverage for certain home visits.[7] Had Bonnie remained in the hospital following her procedure and had she been given access to a support network, her recovery would have been better managed.

To lose a breast is a deeply emotional experience that requires support. When I stood on the floor to drum up support for the bill, I stressed the pain of losing a body part that for many women determines their sexuality and gender. Most women, whether they have a support system at home or not, will be emotional about the loss of a breast. My colleagues understood the need for patients to have proper discharge planning, education, and support. Surprisingly, no one argued against the bill.

CHAPTER 9

Health Care Disparities Prevention

Some of the conditions I encountered as a nurse haunted me. When I was a student at Johns Hopkins University, I took on nursing jobs through a temporary staffing agency and worked in several facilities that needed short-term help, including correctional facilities. Sometimes I worked in nursing homes, where the care the patients received varied from excellent to neglectful. At some homes, the patients didn't receive the proper diet. Some were given solid food even though they didn't have teeth and couldn't chew, which meant their nutritional needs weren't being met. Some facilities were permanently short-staffed, and in these cases the patients were getting bedsores on their backs and ulcers on their heels and urinary tract infections.

As a legislator, I had not forgotten those conditions. I proposed legislation to create a Task Force on Quality of Care in Nursing Homes. Sometimes I think that God was always ahead of me, laying the path when I was doing what he called me to do. This was one of those times. The night before I was scheduled to testify on the bill in the Senate, a television station aired a program on the nightmares in nursing homes. The program showed a patient with a large ulcer on her back. Since the legislation had already passed in the House, I stood up in the Senate Chambers and asked, "Did anyone here see the report last night on the news showing the terrible conditions in Maryland nursing homes?" Several of my colleagues put their hands up.

Senator Bromwell, who was then chair of the Education, Health, and Environmental Affairs Committee, quickly said, "Let's move this bill to a vote."

That legislation passed easily, and its quick movement through the legislative process reminded me of why I had run for office. But I knew, too, that there would be more roadblocks ahead—and, indeed, in 2000, I put forth another bill to address nursing home staffing, another attempt to achieve the right ratio so that patients would be taken care of properly.[1] Care of the elderly was—and continues to be—an ongoing issue.

•

Six years into my new role as a politician, I moved my district office and Nathan's Networks into a new office space. A pharmacy and medical office had moved out of the suite, which was large enough to hold the adult daycare business I had long thought about opening. The daycare was a way to honor my mother and simultaneously provide some means of socialization for elderly and sick patients, especially those like my mother who were disabled from strokes. As a nurse I had visited many stroke patients at home and saw the difficulty families had taking care of the disabled. Often the patients were in homes that had no air conditioning, which can be extremely uncomfortable in Baltimore's hot summers.

It didn't take me long to think about opening the business. Having my district office and the two businesses in the same building would be ideal. The financial aspect, of course, was a bit more challenging. Based on my conversations with the landlord, I would need about $100,000 to prepare the space for the daycare business. Somehow I had to make it work. So I approached banks and private lenders for loans. The interest on the loans, however, would be too high. So I decided to use my own funds. Business gurus generally say that's not the best business practice, but for me, at that time, I thought it was the best way. I borrowed against my savings, took a loan from Nathan's Networks, and negotiated with the landlord to bring the price down. In the end the landlord agreed to knock out the walls, and I would be responsible for the kitchen and the nurses' station. I also negotiated an agreement that I would not have to pay the full rent—over $5,000—at the start of the contract. The landlord agreed to allow me to pay half the rent and add the remainder to the back end of the contract, to repay after I had enough clients and was generating income. I wasn't savvy in real estate negotiations. But a Jamaican friend, Grennett Service, an experienced real estate agent, told me how to negotiate.

I had secured the space and worked out the finances, but setting up the physical business was an even more daunting task. I needed an architect to build out the space to meet the state's specifications, including adding a kitchen, bathrooms with showers, and seating to accommodate all fifty-three clients—the number of clients my business license covered. I needed to establish policies and procedures. I needed to purchase kitchen and laundry appliances, either leather or vinyl seats that staff could easily wipe down, and a van to transport the patients, some of whom would rely on wheelchairs. I needed to hire staff. This business required much more than my first business.

Around that time, I was asked to speak to a group of Nigerian kids at a gathering to celebrate a Nigerian holiday. I was already overwhelmed with all the work I had to do and hesitant about taking time to do another event. But I went to the School of Public Health at Johns Hopkins to meet with the group, and even today I remain grateful that I made the effort. As it turned out, the father of one of the girls in attendance was an architect and artist, Fola. We started talking and I told him about the daycare I planned to open, and my search for an architect to draft plans for the space. He agreed to help, charging me $1,000 then to draft the plans, including building the kitchen as the central gathering place. In any other setting, it would have cost me a lot more. His kindness touched me. We became good friends, and when the daycare was constructed, we displayed much of his artwork there.

Many friends stepped in to help me get the business up and running. Fola and my legislative aide, Sue, both artists, helped me with the color selection. Fola chose colors that brought the light in—burgundy, white, green, and black. My nurse friends, Sarah and Gwen, who had started similar businesses, helped me with policy and procedures manuals. Henry Burris, a retired firefighter, helped me set up the inspection and trained the staff in CPR. Calvin Sadler did the electrical work. My daughter, Sharon, helped with the wallpaper trimming and the kitchen design.

I had budgeted $20,000 for furniture but found out about a business in Jessup that sold surplus furniture, including the furniture that is removed from the State House. My best find was a leather sofa for $50 and chairs for $10 each. I paid a small fee to have the chairs reupholstered. Sue, who worked three days a week in my legislative office, also had a master's degree in art and was willing to work the other two days as the activities coordinator, in charge of creating an activities plan for the patients. Some of her artwork adorned the walls.

Nearly a year after first seeing the available space, I opened Extended Family Adult Medical Daycare Inc. with fifteen patients. A photo of Mama in her wheelchair was prominently placed on the brochures and marketing material—a reminder that caring for my mother after she was disabled by a stroke had been instrumental in starting the business.

Fola's daughter, Adetoun, later asked to join my campaign.

"What do you know about managing a campaign?" I asked.

"Nothing," she said. "But I'm willing to learn."

Adetoun set up my campaign headquarters, and later, when I won reelection, she came to Annapolis as my legislative aide. Today she is an attorney licensed to practice in Maryland and Nigeria.

My experience building and launching the daycare with the help of many friends and acquaintances, and mentoring several young people, reminds me how important it is to build great relationships with good people.

•

Running the adult daycare and the personal care business in Baltimore fed into my work in Annapolis.

I learned from the oral cancer bill and my ultimate decision to remove the racial component in order to get the bill passed that I needed a stronger, more direct approach to address health issues that were worsened by racial inequities. At the federal level, the Office of Minority Health had been in existence since 1986. Created as a result of the landmark *Report of the Secretary's Task Force on Black and Minority Health* (i.e., the *Heckler Report*), the office's mission is to improve the health of racial and ethnic minority populations through developing health policies and programs that will help eliminate health disparities. More specifically, the office funds regional, state, and local programs that contribute to health policy and health-improvement strategies, as well as fosters research, evaluation, data collection, and partnerships to identify and solve health problems.

To get at the heart of the inequities in Maryland, we needed a similar approach. We had the data concerning disparities. In 1985, US Department of Health and Human Services Secretary Margaret Heckler wrote in the *Heckler Report* that American health overall had improved. But "there was a continuing disparity in the burden of death and illness experienced by Blacks and other minority Americans as compared with our nation's population as a whole."[2] The disparity was not new. It had been evident since the federal government began keeping records nearly a generation earlier. And yet, since the report was published in 1985, and despite the recommendations it included, disparities persisted.

In addition, Senator Larry Young had sponsored a bill creating the Governor's Commission on Black and Minority Health. The commission's 1987 report, *Now Is the Time: An Action Agenda for Improving Black and Minority Health in Maryland*, gave an overview of the health status of Blacks and other non-white communities in Maryland and reviewed the factors that contributed to their health experience.[3] The commission focused on several key areas: infant mortality, Black and minority health manpower development, access to primary health care services, and prevention of cardiovascular disease, cancer, mental illness, and AIDS. I served on the mental health subcommittee. The commission also recommended the development of a permanent Governor's Commission on Black and Minority Health to continue the work the commission started. Yet nothing had changed.

Even more recent data showed the persistence of disparities. In 2002, Dr. Brian Smedley, a senior program officer in the Division of Health Sciences Policy of the Institute of Medicine (IOM), coauthored a report on racial and ethnic disparities in health care: *Unequal Treatment: Confronting Racial and Ethnic Disparities in Health Care.*[4] According to the report, racial and ethnic groups generally receive lower-quality health care than white patients, even after factoring in access-related factors, such as patients' insurance status and income. Nationally, the overall health of Americans had improved, yet racial and ethnic groups continued to experience higher rates of morbidity and mortality than white Americans. In particular, African Americans experienced the highest rates of mortality from heart disease, cancer, cerebrovascular disease, and HIV/AIDS than any other racial or ethnic group. Native Americans were more likely to die from diabetes, liver disease, cirrhosis, and unintentional injuries. Among other groups, Hispanic Americans were almost twice as likely as non-Hispanic white persons to die from diabetes. According to the report, the rate at which stomach, liver, and cervical cancers occurred in some Asian American groups was well above national averages.

Access to health insurance and health care could explain some of the disparities. But it was clear that, even with the same level of access to care, racial and ethnic minorities experienced a lower quality of health services and were less likely to receive even routine medical procedures.

Smedley's report underscored the message I had spent years trying to get across to my colleagues: two patients presenting to a medical facility with the same signs and symptoms of cardiac disease do not necessarily get the same treatment. More often than not, the level of care and the treatment approach were lower for Black and poor patients than for white patients.

Several years before Smedley's study was published, I had learned this directly. Late one night in 1997, I went to a Baltimore area emergency room with shortness of breath and wheezing. The medical staff performed a series of tests but could find nothing wrong. Finally, the female doctor attending to me said, "I am sure you, a busy legislator and RN, would not be here if these symptoms weren't real. So I'm going to bring in the on-call radiologist."

Having had rheumatic fever as a child, I had lingering cardiac issues. I had spent a lifetime monitoring changes in my body. I saw a cardiologist regularly. Armed also with the knowledge I had gained over the years as a nurse, I knew something was not right. I waited for the radiologist to arrive, mulling over my symptoms and what they could point to.

When the radiologist got to the room, the staff proceeded with a cardiac catheterization, a procedure used to diagnose and treat cardiovascular conditions. The radiologist inserted a catheter in an artery in my groin and threaded it through my blood vessels to my heart. In my lungs was an embolism—an obstruction of an artery, sometimes caused by a blood clot or an air bubble, which can be fatal. I was immediately transferred from the emergency room to the intensive care unit and quickly treated with anticoagulant medications and put under cardiac monitoring.

But the sobering fact was what the doctor had said about my occupation. She believed my symptoms were serious simply because I was a registered nurse and legislator. Had the doctor not recognized me or known my occupation, I may not have been treated at all. I would have been sent home, and quite likely would have died undiagnosed and untreated. The bias was clear. There were too many others who looked like me who had not been so lucky.

Years later I would learn of another Black woman who presented to the hospital with similar symptoms as mine but with a vastly different outcome. In September 2011, Anna Brown, a homeless woman living in St. Louis, visited two hospitals with severe leg pain after spraining her ankle. The twenty-nine-year-old mother was examined and discharged from both hospitals when the medical staff found no reason for her severe pain. Brown visited a third hospital, where she was again examined and discharged. This time she refused to leave. The hospital staff called the police, who arrested her for trespassing. She died in police custody, and an autopsy later revealed that blood clots that had started in her legs had traveled to her lungs, causing her death.

Anna Brown died from a treatable condition because she didn't get the proper care she deserved. Had it not been for my occupation, I could have suffered the same fate. Understanding and addressing disparities in health care could lead to fewer stories like these. No doubt implicit bias—the thoughts and feelings that often exist outside of conscious awareness—played a role in our cases. I was "believable" because I fit the doctor's perceptions of a nurse and legislator. Anna Brown fit another perception altogether, and this bias took her life.

•

From my experience, my fellow legislators had little interest in understanding the root causes of disparities. A few years before I won my first election and became a delegate, I was invited to serve on a task force to study heart disease, the treatments in white and Black populations, and why the death rate from cardiovascular disease was higher among Black men than white men. As a group we began probing why white men presenting with symptoms indicative of cardiovascular disease were given scans and catheterization, which saved their lives. Black men, on the other hand, were not given similar advanced treatment options. Before we could fully understand the issues, the task force was disbanded without explanation.

The termination of the task force pointed to a general lack of interest in fully understanding the disparities and taking remedial steps. After being elected, I started the Congress on Health and Economic Disparities (CHED) to bring knowledgeable health professionals together to serve as a sounding board on racial and economic disparities and to give advice on the legislations I presented. They were invaluable, reviewing bills and suggesting improvements.

By 2003, as a member of the General Assembly, I knew I had to take more direct action to ensure that treatment was equal across racial and ethnic groups, and that there were ongoing opportunities to educate my colleagues and the community on racial disparities. The long-term goal was still racial health equity, but reaching that goal required a greater understanding of disparities.

In the 2003 session, I proposed the Health Care Services Disparities Prevention Act, requiring the Department of Health and other entities to develop and implement a plan over the following five years to reduce health care disparities based on gender, race, ethnicity, and poverty.[5] The legislation targeted education through courses and seminars that addressed how health care practitioners identified and eliminated health care services disparities of minority populations.

One year later, I followed up with another piece of legislation to establish the Maryland Office of Minority Health and Health Disparities (OMH) within the Maryland Department of Health. The office promotes health and prevention of disease among African Americans, Hispanics, Asian and Pacific Islanders, and Native Americans and provides grants for improving minority health and health disparities.[6] Getting this legislation passed was no easy feat. The primary issue standing in the way was lack of funding for such an office. Had it not been for various institutions, such as Johns Hopkins University School of Nursing, the University of Maryland School of Medicine, and Morgan State University, all promising to provide in-kind contributions, such as note-taking and administrative support if needed, the legislation would not have passed. I worked hard to have the bill placed in statute, meaning that future administrations could not close the office without going through the legislative process.

Around that time, I had a conversation with Delegate Pete Rawlings, who was then chair of the Appropriations Committee. I wanted to know what portion of the Cigarette Restitution Fund would go directly to the Black community. I reminded him that the tobacco companies advertised heavily in Black communities, and cigarettes they promoted to the Black communities had a high concentration of nicotine and tar, both known to cause cardiovascular disease and cancers, which affected the state's Black communities at a high rate. Following that conversation, more funds were directed to those communities.

After the legislation was passed, Dr. Carlessia A. Hussein, then director of the Cigarette Restitution Fund, was named head of the Office of Minority Health. Running both offices gave her the flexibility to use some of the funds from the Cigarette Restitution Fund to create the Minority Outreach and Technical Assistance program in fifteen counties. She gave small grants in these counties to conduct a range of smoking cessation programs aimed at reducing cancer mortality, as well as pregnancy navigator programs to reduce infant mortality and low birth weight. Later studies showed that the minority outreach programs and the smoking cessation program led to a reduction in cancer rates.

•

When I first moved to Baltimore, Sinai Hospital—which was founded in 1866 as a ten-room hospital for the needs of Jewish patients and doctors—served a predominantly white population. Today, the Park Heights neighborhood, where Sinai Hospital is located, is a different place. Park Heights is home to a significant number of Jamaicans and other Caribbean immigrants, and the once-thriving community is a shell of what it once was. Though the culture of Park Heights had changed over the years, Sinai's medical personnel had not kept up with the customs brought by this new influx of immigrants. Though diabetes and high blood pressure occurred at high rates in the Caribbean immigrant communities, doctors didn't necessarily know the types of foods the Caribbean immigrants ate. Without knowledge of the specific foods in a patient's diet, a doctor or nurse counseling a diabetic Caribbean patient to reduce starchy foods would not necessarily know that the patient would return home to eat fried or boiled plantain, yam and sweet potatoes, or rice and peas—all foods that the body converts to sugar. The doctor or nurse would not necessarily know that the Jamaican patient also prepared rice and peas with coconut milk, which contributed additional fat. Without those details, the dietary counseling would never be adequate.

As a nursing student, I had studied cultural competency, and when I had worked on the floor, those lessons had helped me determine which patients to place near the nursing station. In some cultures, pain is something to grin and bear, and in others the patient learns early to vocalize pain and discomfort and ask for relief. That knowledge helped me know which surgical patients I had to monitor more closely and check for clammy skin because they would never ask for pain medicine.

Cultural competency—the ability of doctors and other health practitioners to recognize individuals' cultural beliefs, values, attitudes, traditions, language preferences, and health practices and apply this knowledge to influence positive health outcomes—was an important part of achieving health equity. Decades of work in health care services had taught me that some of the disparities in the treatment patients received were tied to providers' lack of awareness of the customs and cultural practices of their patients.

Taking steps to increase health care providers' understanding and appreciation of cultural differences among Maryland residents could affect the outcomes of certain diseases. In 2006, I proposed a bill requiring the Department of Health's Family Health Administration to work with the OMH to develop a pilot program that addressed the cultural competency training of health care providers.[7] The bill also set goals for specific diseases, including improvement of body mass index and hemoglobin A1C levels for diabetics, improvement in blood pressure, hypertension, and cholesterol levels for individuals with cardiac disease, and increased cancer screening for prostate, breast, and cervical cancers.

I wanted to ensure that the underserved populations benefited from the program. The bill required that the program be implemented in a state-based community teaching hospital that served a medically underserved area and medically underserved populations.

Two years later, I sponsored another bill requiring higher educational institutions with programs in medicine, nursing, pharmacy, and dentistry in Maryland to report to the OMH and certain legislative committees on courses that they developed independently or through collaboration with the Office of Minority Health and Health Disparities. And in 2017, I sponsored similar legislation requiring each health occupations board established under the Health Occupations Article to report on their efforts to educate certain health care professionals regarding racial and ethnic health disparities.

Despite the initial objections to the cultural competency requirements, medical and nursing schools have begun to teach courses and incorporate cultural competency in their curriculum. Above all, I knew the OMH would remain the central place through which all corrective actions, like cultural competency training, would be monitored. That office would follow through on the lessons resulting from years of studies and experience about health care inequities. Recently, though, the office has been weakened. While it is still operating, it isn't sufficiently funded and staffed, making it impossible to consistently execute its mission. The weakening of the office is typical of what happens to programs that address health disparities. I have hope that this office will rise like a phoenix to accomplish my dreams of full equity.

•

I wondered whether other countries dealt with disparities similar to those found in America. In 2005, when I learned about a trip to Cuba planned by health care professionals in Baltimore (and approved by the State Department), I asked to join the group, which included former Baltimore City and Howard County health commissioner Dr. Peter Beilenson, Johns Hopkins pediatrician Dr. George Dover, and University of Maryland surgeon Dr. Stephen Bartlett, among others. I was impressed by the health care delivery system, especially since Cuba did not have the resources the United States had. Health care delivery included a dedicated doctor, nurse, and social worker who tended to the needs of the residents in a specific province. If a resident was too sick to travel to the medical facility, the medical providers visited the patient at home, and if the patient required hospitalization, the medical provider accompanied the patient to the hospital. Medication was provided at no cost. Additionally, Cuba trained doctors from different countries—even with its limited resources. I came back to America knowing we could do better to address health disparities here.

That is not to say we hadn't tried to address the issue on a national level. We had. One approach was the National Partnership for Action to End Health Disparities established by the OMH, headed by Jamaican-born Garth Graham, MD, who was the Assistant Secretary of Health, the director for the OMH, and responsible for implementing the National Partnership for Action to End Health Disparities. OMH set out to build a national, comprehensive, community-based and -sustained approach to health disparities, as well as move toward health equity. OMH's approach included a national summit of nearly 2,000 leaders who were tasked with developing tactics to reduce health disparities and advance health equity. I served on the task force, which produced the *National Stakeholder Strategy for Achieving Health Equity* report. The report provides an overarching road map for eliminating health disparities through cooperative and strategic actions.[8] Through that experience, I gained tremendous insight into the needs of Black and brown people, as well as the historical and contemporary injustices that continued to fuel health disparities. Being a part of those meetings made clear that achieving health equity was not possible without health equality.

CHAPTER 10

Affordable Health Insurance for All

The cheers from the crowd at Invesco Field were steady on that August day in 2008 when we gathered in Denver, Colorado, to officially nominate Barack Obama as the Democratic Party's presidential nominee. Outside, the rain was heavy and steady, matching the overwhelming feeling of exuberance and anticipation that filled the stadium. For me, the magnitude of the moment and of the Democratic Party electing the first Black man for the highest office in America was captured most clearly in the energy and enthusiasm of a centenarian who had traveled from Tuskegee, Alabama, to be part of the festivities.

I had been attending the Democratic National Conventions since the 1992 event in New York City and later went on to serve at the 1996 convention in Chicago, Illinois, as an elected delegate for the reelection of President Bill Clinton and Vice President Al Gore. Each state chooses delegates to represent their state at their party's national nominating convention. Delegates are often party activists, local political leaders, or early supporters of a presidential candidate and are selected in primaries, caucuses, or local party conventions. I had long been involved in the Democratic Central Committee, my first elected office since 1990. As a delegate, I sat up front with Senator Barbara Mikulski, Senator Sarbanes, then congressman Ben Cardin, and other members of the Maryland Delegation.

In 2000, I attended the convention in Los Angeles when Al Gore was the nominee and again in 2004, in Boston when John Kerry was the nominee. That year, the most exciting part was Barack Obama delivering the mesmerizing, inspiring speech that launched him on to the national scene. Everyone was absolutely blown away by his charisma and passion, and in 2008, I was looking forward to seeing him captivate the audience as he had done years earlier.

In 2008, I was not a delegate, but years of attending conventions had taught me a few lessons, including how to network to secure passes to get on the floor, how to get close seats, and what shoes to wear. When I attended my first convention, in New York City, Louis Goldstein, then comptroller of Maryland, advised everyone to wear comfortable shoes, but I wanted to be dressed to the nines, as they say, so I wore high heels. Even now I remember walking the long city blocks to get to the receptions and parties, and developing blisters. With each step all I wanted to do was take off my shoes and walk the rest of the way in my stockings.

I also learned how information filters from the convention to constituents back home. In New York, a young man dressed up like a painter had wandered the halls drawing caricatures of anyone who wanted one. He approached me and asked where I wanted my painting placed. I was wearing a low-cut dress and asked him to paint a heart and arrow right above my cleavage. Later that evening a gentleman approached me and said, "Committeewoman, are you having fun here in New York?"

"Yes," I said.

"How are you having fun?"

"I am having my cleavage painted," I said.

Back home, after the Sunday church service, I went to shake our minister's hand. Father Cantler asked me, "What were you doing in New York having your cleavage painted?"

I was shocked. "How do you know that?"

Father Cantler had read Barry Rascovar's column in the *Baltimore Sun*, in which he asked various attendees what they were doing for fun. Most politicians told him about visiting museums, shopping, or sightseeing, but the most memorable response was mine: having my cleavage painted.

I learned that I needed to pay closer attention to what I said and to whom I spoke.

I used those age-old lessons to maneuver my way around the convention. I was excited for this convention and the opportunity to see Barack Obama. That night in 2008 when Barack Obama took the stage in Denver, I was so excited to see him light up the stage on the final night of the convention and proud to be an active member of the Maryland delegation. Here was a man who looked like me, standing before a crowd of thousands to accept the nomination to run for the highest office in America.

I had met the future president once before at a reception for his first book, *Dreams from My Father: A Story of Race and Inheritance*, when he was still a senator. At the reception in downtown Baltimore for elected officials, I got two books—one for my friend Alice Torriente and another for myself. I remember telling him that Alice was crazy about him and his wife, Michelle. Then-senator Obama signed the book for Alice, but as he was about to sign mine, his security team swept in because he had to leave. When it was clear that he would receive the nomination for presidency, I jokingly asked Alice for the signed book. "Oh, no," she said. "This book says 'to Alice.'"

In the early stages of the democratic campaign, I had supported Hillary Clinton and even campaigned for her. On one occasion, I shared a stage with Hillary Clinton's mother, who had come to Annapolis to campaign on her daughter's behalf. But I was also struck by the young Black man who campaigned hard, gathered a significant following, and raised millions of dollars in a very short time. My granddaughter, Jaye-Ann, who was still a teenager, was a strong supporter of Barack Obama. I switched my allegiance to Obama. I was devoted to getting him elected as our first African American president.

When he took the stage that day, everyone paid attention, lapping up his every word. He was as mesmerizing as I remembered.

"Now is the time to finally keep the promise of affordable, accessible health care for every single American," he told the crowd in the packed convention center.

I nodded and cheered, along with everyone else. Here was a man, addressing the concerns I'd had when I met Stella so many years earlier.

Obama laid out his vision. "For over two decades, [Senator McCain has] subscribed to that old, discredited Republican philosophy—give more and more to those with the most and hope that prosperity trickles down to everyone else. In Washington, they call this the Ownership Society, but what it really means is—you are on your own. Out of work? Tough luck. No health care? The market will fix it. Born into poverty? Pull yourself up by your own bootstraps—even if you don't have boots. You're on your own."

Obama's words mirrored what I had seen and what I had been fighting for as an elected official in Maryland. For the entirety of my political career, I ran on these issues. My campaign theme was the "nurse for your political health." I looked at every aspect of health. Most people say education is the number one priority, but I have long believed that health is the first and foremost priority and what centers everything else. A person who is not healthy—whether physically or emotionally—will have a hard time achieving his or her goals. I have long looked at the ability to achieve education and financial goals through the equity lens.

I left the convention feeling renewed and hopeful that America could revamp the health care system that had failed so many, especially the working poor who often hold several jobs at one time to make ends meet. These jobs often don't offer health insurance, and with an income, the working poor usually make just about enough to prevent them from accessing subsidized health care. Of course, I remembered Stella and so many others like her whose diagnoses were delayed or prevented because they lacked health care. That was one piece of the health care crisis I hoped the Obama administration could change.

•

Six months into President Obama's first term, a group of Democrats from the House of Representatives, including Speaker of the House

Nancy Pelosi, revealed the Affordable Health Care for America Act, their plan for overhauling the health care system. At its core was a plan to create a system through which all Americans could purchase health insurance regardless of employment status and preexisting conditions—two primary roadblocks to obtaining insurance.

I sprang into action. At that time, I chaired the Minority Health Disparities Subcommittee of the Health and Government Operations Committee in Maryland's House of Delegates (a position I held until 2014 when I won a seat in the Maryland Senate). I cohosted town hall meetings to lobby for inclusion of the option to purchase public health insurance. The public option, as it was called, would reduce overall health care costs and save the federal government money. Most of the savings would be generated from one of two things: a subsidy reduction or a tax base increase. The public option, however, was one of the most contentious issues in the debate over the plan.

Fredette West, founder and then director of the African American Health Alliance (AAHA) and cofounder and chair of the Racial and Ethnic Health Disparities Coalition (REHDC), came to me with the idea to add an amendment to the proposal that would lead to greater consideration of racial and ethnic disparities at the federal level. We brought Dr. Carlessia Hussein, director of the Office of Minority Health, into the conversation and put our heads together to figure out how best to approach the plan to elevate the existing offices of minority health at the federal level to a new designation: Center of Excellence. We understood that the key to increasing awareness of racial disparities was elevating the offices of minority health within federal agencies to centers and strengthening their eligibility to receive a larger portion of grant money. Elevating these offices ensured greater attention to the very real concerns of how health and racial disparities affect access to and quality of care.

Almost immediately, we ran into roadblocks. Senator Ted Kennedy, who had spent much of his career on efforts to ensure all Americans had access to the same quality of health care services he could access as a senator, had just been diagnosed with a brain tumor. Moreover, his staff was reluctant to add our amendment to an already long bill. We went to the staff of Senator Harry Reid, who was then Senate Majority Leader; they turned us down, again because of the length of the bill. We approached Maryland Senator Ben Cardin's office and received the same response. Our options were dwindling.

Weeks later, Senator Cardin held a health committee meeting in Towson, Maryland. Near the end of the program, I raised my hand. "Senator Cardin," I said, "are you and Senator Barbara Mikulski aware of the morbidity and mortality rates and racial and ethnic health disparities of Blacks in Maryland?"

"Yes," he said. "Let's talk after this meeting."

There was a line of people waiting to ask questions, but I waited patiently to tell him about the amendment we wanted to add to the Affordable Care Act (ACA). That conversation paved the way for further discussions with his staff. Several staff members were in the room that day, including the senator's policy director, Priscilla, whom we had previously approached regarding the amendment.

"We really need your help," I said. She promised to do whatever she could.

The size of the legislation remained our biggest obstacle. Fredette made many trips to Capitol Hill to trim the amendment so it could get in. At last, the amendment was incorporated into the management section of the ACA.

The amendment elevated eight federal offices on minority health at several agencies to the Center of Excellence:

- Agency for Healthcare Research and Quality (AHRQ)
- Centers for Disease Control and Prevention (CDC)
- Centers for Medicare and Medicaid Services (CMS)
- Food and Drug Administration (FDA)
- Health Resources and Services Administration (HRSA)
- National Institutes of Health (NIH)

- Office of Minority Health (OMH) at the US Department of Health and Human Services
- Substance Abuse and Mental Health Services Administration (SAMHSA)

Before the legislation passed, the NIH was operating a Center for Health Disparities. After the bill passed, the center was elevated to an institute—the National Institute on Minority Health and Health Disparities—which meant it was given access to increased grants to address critical issues with health disparities.

•

Despite continued efforts to weaken and invalidate the ACA, studies show that coverage under the legislation has reduced racial and ethnic disparities in health coverage rates. While all racial and ethnic groups saw gains, health coverage for individuals from low-income groups also improved, especially in states that participated in the Medicaid expansion. Across Maryland, the decline in the number of uninsured people told a story of the legislation's importance. Three years after President Obama signed the ACA into law, Maryland began to see the uninsured rate dropping across the state. Between 2013 and 2016, the number of uninsured individuals in Maryland declined from 593,000 to 363,000, or 38.8 percent. Nationally, the decline in the uninsured rate was similarly impressive. Between 2013 and 2014, the number of uninsured individuals declined from 45 million to 36.7 million people, or 18.8 percent. By 2016, six years after the legislation was passed into law, the national uninsured rate was about 8.6 percent versus 16.3 percent in 2010, 14.5 percent in 2013, and 11.7 percent in 2014.[1]

Nationwide, the ACA improved health insurance coverage for white, Black, and Hispanic adults. Data from the American Community Survey and the *American Journal of Public Health* show that the ACA reduced racial and ethnic disparities in coverage. In 2013, 40.5 percent of Hispanics and 25.8 percent of Black Americans were uninsured, compared with 14.8 percent of white Americans. Data from 2014 following the implementation of the primary provisions of the health insurance law show that coverage disparities declined slightly. The percentage of uninsured Hispanic adults decreased by 7.1 percentage points, 5.1 percentage points for Black Americans, and 3 percentage points for white Americans. In addition, the gains in coverage gains were greater in states, like Maryland, that expanded Medicaid programs.[2]

Gains were again seen in 2015. Analysis from the Urban Institute shows that about 19.2 million nonelderly people gained health insurance coverage from 2010 to 2015, following implementation of the ACA. The gains in coverage were seen across all racial and ethnic groups and educational levels. In addition, about 2.8 million children through age eighteen gained coverage. Nationally, the number of uninsured adults between ages nineteen and thirty-four declined by 8.7 million or 42 percent, while the number of uninsured adults ages thirty-five to fifty-four declined by 5.6 million or 33 percent. Through the same time period, another 2 million adults ages fifty-five to sixty-four obtained coverage under the law. From the perspective of race, 8.2 million or 43 percent of those gaining coverage were non-Hispanic white, 2.8 million or 15 percent were non-Hispanic Black, 6.2 million or 32 percent were Hispanic, and 2 million or 10 percent were other non-Hispanics. The study also found that 87 percent of adults gaining coverage in that time period did not have a college degree.[3]

The ACA, while not perfect, created opportunities to level the playing field for many Americans who had no or limited access to affordable health care. This imperfect law was better than nothing, and certainly better than the system under which this country had long operated. Back when the law was passed, and even now, I think about what a law of this kind would have meant for Stella. Surely, subsidized health care similar to the type the ACA provides would have given Stella earlier access to health care and would have reduced or eliminated the burden of waiting to get a job to get health insurance. The benefits would have gone beyond access to coverage. The ACA provides preventive care, such as screening mammograms and colonoscopies, at no cost to patients. It also removes barriers like yearly and lifetime dollar limits on the amount of coverage a health plan pays for and prevents health plans from charging more to clients who have preexisting conditions or refusing coverage for those clients. The law spelled out specific coverage pertaining to breast cancer. All of this would have helped Stella. Private individual and group insurance plans must cover the full cost of mammograms starting at age forty, genetic screening for high-risk women, and breast cancer preventive medication for high-risk women. In states that expanded Medicaid coverage under the ACA, women are allowed the same screening and preventive services as those provided to women via private insurance.

I imagine an entirely different scenario—Stella having health coverage independent of her employment status, seeking routine care as soon as she suspected something was wrong, and a doctor catching the lump in her breast long before it grew to the size I felt in the hospital that day. I imagine her getting early treatment and going on to live the life she had planned. Perhaps the story I tell about Stella today would have been a different one.

CHAPTER 11

How Government Policies Sometimes Fuel Disparities

"Joe died."

I don't remember the time of day the call came in or which of Joe's relatives called, but I remember the despair I felt and the heartbreak, then and even now. Joe had been working as a driver for one of my businesses for nearly fifteen years when he died. He picked up patients and transported them to the adult day care center and to medical appointments. For some time, my son, Wayne, who was the chief operating officer of Extended Family Adult Medical Day Care, had been telling me that Joe wasn't well. At that time I didn't know the extent of Joe's condition.

"It's looking worse, Mom," Wayne said one day.

I carved out time from my already overbooked schedule and went by the office trying to catch Joe as he came in to begin his shift. When Joe arrived, I called him into the office and looked him over. Something was indeed very wrong.

"You need to see a doctor today," I told him, and offered to go with him.

Joe agreed.

I called the University of Maryland Medical Center myself and spoke with the president of the hospital system with whom I had a working relationship. After I relayed what I was looking for, the president, in turn, called Dr. Stewart, an internist, who was able to see Joe that day. We stopped by Joe's house to retrieve all his recent medical records he had on hand and headed to the doctor's office at the University of Maryland.

I drove us there, and as I was parking, Joe hopped out, ready to cross the street alone.

"No, no, I am going in with you," I said. I wanted to make sure he was seen. Given how weak he was, I had to help him undress.

The doctor looked through Joe's medical records, specifically his previous bloodwork, and said he suspected Joe had cancer of some kind. The diagnosis was heartbreaking, the news doubly disconcerting because the cause of Joe's problems was clearly laid out in the paperwork he had in his possession. But Joe had been getting health care at a free medical clinic, where he had been getting treatment long before he came to work with me, and the medical clinic staff had not been reviewing the results to see what was causing Joe's symptoms. Joe had health insurance through my company and could have sought help elsewhere. Instead, he continued to see practitioners at the overworked clinic that didn't offer the continuity of care he would have received from a primary care physician.

Joe's situation was grave. The doctor ordered additional blood tests and scans, and subsequently diagnosed Joe with hepatitis C and cancer of the liver. Almost immediately, Joe started chemotherapy. But he was living alone in Baltimore, away from his family in North Carolina, and had no one to care for him. When I visited Joe at the University of Maryland Medical Center, his eyes followed me as if to say, "Say it ain't so."

That was the last time I saw him.

His adult daughter moved him back to North Carolina to live with family there. Within three months of his diagnosis, he was dead.

•

By the time Joe died in 2012, hepatitis C—a disease dubbed the silent killer because patients typically don't know they have it until irreversible liver damage has already occurred—was a disease I had been fighting to get funding for, with little success. Roughly 4.5 million persons in the United States were infected with hepatitis C in 2003, with about 12,000 people dying each year from the disease. Deaths attributed to hepatitis C increased to 17,253 in 2017, according to the CDC.[1] And an estimated 2.4 million people in the United States were living with hepatitis C during 2013 to 2016. In addition to patients who received blood transfusions and solid organ transplants before July 1992, when testing of blood donors improved, those at high risk for hepatitis C infection include current and former drug users, patients with HIV infection, chronic hemodialysis patients, health care workers and first responders, and children born to mothers with hepatitis C.

Developing more serious complications from hepatitis C infection is a real possibility for a large percentage of patients infected with the virus. Of every one hundred people infected with the hepatitis C virus, about five to twenty-five of them will develop cirrhosis within a ten-to-twenty-year period. Those patients who develop cirrhosis are at risk of developing cancer and progressive deterioration in liver function. Patients more likely to develop cirrhosis after becoming infected with the hepatitis C virus are likely to be males over fifty years; those who consume alcohol; those with nonalcoholic fatty liver disease, hepatitis B, or HIV coinfection; and those receiving immunosuppressive therapy.

At the federal level, the Department of Health and Human Services implemented a plan to address hepatitis C, including taking steps to identify and notify the individuals who were inadvertently infected through blood transfusions. Without a vaccine, educating individuals at high risk for hepatitis C and taking steps to prevent its spread was of utmost importance.

For nearly fifteen years, I submitted different versions of legislation to tackle hepatitis C infections, but time and time again I met resistance, often because of the projected cost. The drugs were expensive, and the potential cost of the bill was a major concern to the legislators who refused to support it.

In 2003, I proposed a bill establishing a State Advisory Council on Hepatitis C to review, recommend changes to, and solicit funds to implement a specified hepatitis C prevention plan.[2] My attempts to get funds for hepatitis infections were not limited to hepatitis C. In 2001, I sponsored a House Joint Resolution concerning federal funding for a hepatitis B vaccination program. That plan urged the Secretary of Health and Mental Hygiene to seek federal funds to offset the cost to the state of providing the vaccines. At the time, Maryland had an infection rate for hepatitis A—which is usually caused by contaminated food—ranging from 5 to 10 cases per 100,000 in the northern and western parts of the state to more than 20 cases per 100,000 in the metropolitan Baltimore area.

Two other attempts to create a hepatitis A, B, and C education and prevention program failed in the 2001 and 2002 sessions.

But hepatitis C was more deadly than hepatitis A and B, and without a concrete plan, the rate of infections would only continue to increase. The State Advisory Council's first report on the state of hepatitis C in Maryland issued in January 2006 showed us that, while efforts to make hepatitis C infection reportable by medical laboratories and health care providers had increased the ability to assess Maryland's burden of hepatitis C, about two-thirds of the cases in the state were still unreported.[3] We also learned that the resources were not adequate to meet the needs of local health departments, especially in some densely populated areas.

In 1980, Maryland had begun requiring health care providers to report hepatitis C infections—then called "hepatitis, type non-A, non-B," before being renamed "hepatitis C" in 2003. It was not until 2001 that medical laboratories were required to report laboratory evidence of hepatitis C infection. Even with the limited data, I knew we had a significant problem we needed to address. Based on data reported to the Maryland Electronic Reporting and Surveillance System (MERSS)—the Maryland Department of Health's communicable disease database—about 26,000 cases of hepatitis C infection were reported between 2001 and 2004. About 63 percent of the infected patients were male. Where race was reported, 54 percent of the patients were white and 44 percent were African American. There was no data on race, however, for nearly half the patients.

One of the most pressing roadblocks to measuring problems that would help determine the burden of hepatitis C in Maryland was that 80 percent of individuals had no easily recognizable symptoms, which meant infected patients were often diagnosed only when the disease had already caused significant harm. The state's own approach to treating hepatitis C, particularly among inmates, was also a contributing factor in the continuing increase in Maryland's hepatitis C infection rates. At one point, the prison system treated only a fraction of the infected prisoners, opting to treat only those whose sentences were longer than the treatment course. The prison system reasoned that inmates released before the treatment ended would not finish the course of treatment after they were released. So those patients were not treated at all and once released likely went home to infect their sexual partners. The early versions of the treatment drugs had a lot of side effects, and there was wide concern that the side effects would limit the number of patients who complied with the full treatment plan.

Maryland had a significant problem that would only continue to get worse without meaningful intervention.

•

Three years later, in 2015, I introduced another bill related to hepatitis C. The bill required the Department of Health to conduct needs assessment, implement a public awareness campaign, and coordinate with certain units of state government to activate a hepatitis C virus plan. That proposal got nowhere; it did not even come up for a vote in committee.

By 2006, pharmaceutical companies had developed a treatment that cured a subset of hepatitis C patients. But those treatments, while effective in some patients, required a yearlong commitment. One side effect was flu-like symptoms for the entire course of treatment. As a result, medical providers carefully screened patients to determine who would best benefit from it. Over time, drug manufacturers developed another treatment that cured patients within three months and had fewer side effects. Yet because of the high costs, Maryland's Medicaid program covered treatment only for patients with significant liver damage. On the other hand, the nonfinancial costs of not treating hepatitis C patients was also high. Not only was the rate of infection continuing to rise as infected patients passed it to others, but morally we were failing a subset of the population. By not treating all hepatitis C patients with an effective and available cure, the state was contributing to and maintaining health disparities among Maryland's poorest residents.

In committee meeting after committee meeting, I pushed for equitable treatment of all Marylanders infected with hepatitis C. I talked about how hepatitis C spreads through semen and blood, similar to the way HIV is spread. Without treatment, the disease would continue to spread, especially in the most vulnerable populations and among persons who had intimate contact with men and women returning from prison.

But despite that knowledge and the potential for the cost of the drug to decline over time, the early bills I put in failed to gain traction. It took three tries before the bill mandating parity in treatment for all persons infected with hepatitis C passed. One piece of legislation went down in committee, despite a hard-fought battle. Another was drafted but didn't move beyond that stage, in part because of the cost of the bill and resistance from a local medical group, Maryland State Medical Society (MedChi). One point of contention with the second bill was a requirement that doctors ask patients born between 1945 and 1965 if they wanted to be tested for hepatitis C. Patients who fell in that age range were more likely to be positive at that time given the sexual practices of the Woodstock era. But some medical groups were concerned that doctors might face lawsuits if they forgot to test those patients. Groups like the National Medical Association, however, which comprises black doctors, supported the bill, as well as research physicians from Johns Hopkins Hospital and doctors from Health Care for the Homeless. Health Care for the Homeless receives a large percentage of patients released from prison and as the health care provider for these former inmates was well aware of the prevalence and devastating effects of hepatitis C in this population. All these medical providers supporting the bill understood that a large percentage of people infected with hepatitis C and returning from the prison system were Black men.

Once again the bill died. Not until 2019, with support from the American Civil Liberties Union (ACLU) of Maryland, did the Assembly pass a bill that required the Maryland Medical Assistance Program to cover drugs for the treatment of hepatitis C, regardless of a patient's fibrosis score or the progress of the disease.[4] In January 2018, the ACLU of Maryland stated that it would pursue legal action concerning Maryland Medicaid criteria for patients who can receive hepatitis C therapies. The ACLU had brought suits in other states. Like me, the ACLU thought the policy of treating only some patients was immoral and would lead to disastrous public health consequences. Getting the legislation passed took a lot of work with fiscal services, the state health department, and federal government agencies to get the $33.3 million in funding from a variety of sources. Of the total, $10.5 million was supported by the governor and came from the state's general funds, and $18.5 million came from federal funds. That amount covered Medicaid patients with a Metavir score between 1 and 4. But I wanted to make sure that the Metavir scoring system, which is used to assess the extent of inflammation and fibrosis in patients with hepatitis C, was eliminated. The Metavir grade indicates the activity or degree of inflammation while the stage represents the amount of fibrosis or scarring. To eliminate the score, we needed an additional $4 million, which came from state and federal funds. As a result, all Medicaid patients with hepatitis C are treated regardless of the extent of their liver damage.

I came out of this fight thinking that lawmakers should be penalized when they have all the facts about an issue, particularly a dangerous health concern like hepatitis C, and deliberately vote against legislation that can address that issue and save lives. Long before the bill was passed, state legislators and the administration knew the dangers of hepatitis C, knew it could be treated, knew treatment would save lives and prevent needless spread. This fight for equity in the treatment of hepatitis C showed me again and again that it is easier to get legislation passed when legislators are personally affected.

Throughout the years, each time I get angry that we're not doing enough to address health disparities, I return to Claude McKay's "The Negro's Tragedy." McKay, a Jamaican-born poet, lived during the Harlem Renaissance. The words of the poem rejuvenate me and remind me why I served as a legislator, what I worked toward, and whom I worked for:

It is the Negro's tragedy I feel
Which binds me like a heavy iron chain.
It is the Negro's wounds I want to heal
Because I know the keenness of his pain.

CHAPTER 12

Education Equity Is Health Equity

When I was a delegate in the House, a group of children from the Odyssey School for students with dyslexia and language learning deficiencies came to Annapolis to testify in support of a grant the school sought. Groups and individuals from communities of all kinds often came to provide support for legislation underway or causes they wanted legislators to support. As a dyslexic person who had struggled to learn in traditional educational settings, I was eager to hear from this group of children.

One by one the students told stories about their learning differences—their inability to tell the letter "b" from the letter "d"; how they mixed up "m" and "n"; how they sometimes read backward. The more the children talked, the more my eyes welled with tears. I was reliving my childhood and the frustrations I felt as a child who had the same reading and arithmetic problems they described. As a nurse with multiple tertiary degrees and a legislator, I had already accomplished more than I could have imagined, yet all the frustrations, fears, and shame from my childhood were still inside me rising to the surface. I was so overcome by their stories, I had to step outside to compose myself. When I returned, I told them that I, too, had dyslexia. Later, after I was elected to the Senate, the Decoding Dyslexia group brought children to testify. I heard their stories and had the same reaction that I had in the House. I began to cry. The memory of all I had suffered as a child resurfaced.

I was amazed that the students at the Odyssey School had a community of educators who understood their learning differences and were committed to seeing them thrive. As a child growing up in Jamaica, my parents and teachers did not understand that I learned differently. I struggled under the weight of their expectations, trying to learn multiplication tables, figure out math problems at the board while the class looked on at my mistakes, or answer my father's questions at the dining table. What was also stunning was the difference between the resources available to the Odyssey School children and the resources I had had as a young mother in the 1970s trying to parent a dyslexic child.

Unlike these children before me, figuring out the cause of my own learning issues didn't come until much later in my life. I did not have a name for my own learning challenges until I was already a young adult studying nursing in England. I found out the name by accident and not because I was tested. Because I had rheumatic fever as a child, I had lingering cardiac issues and often needed medical care. In England, my primary care doctor also served as my cardiologist. That was a different time when doctors still made house calls to attend to sick patients. We developed a strong relationship and often talked about concerns and issues outside my immediate medical issues. On one of those home visits, I talked about my challenges studying and distinguishing certain letters when I read material for school. I had accepted the challenge to attend nursing school, but learning the apothecary and the metric systems and studying formulas to calculate medications was hard for me. Miscalculating medications because of my difficulty with numbers was one of my great fears. So on examinations in particular, I took great care going over my calculations. When most students finished their exams and left the room, I remained checking and rechecking to make sure I had not miscalculated numbers. I told the doctor my fears. She listened and started putting together all the learning problems I described.

"Do you know you're dyslexic?" she asked.

Finally, I had a name for this challenge that I had lived with for so long and fought to overcome. I wasn't lazy or unmotivated as the adults in my life once thought. I wasn't dumb as my father had said. I learned differently. Being able to name what was at the root of my learning difficulties brought a little relief.

Dyslexia, I would later learn, is not simply the inability to recognize certain letters but a language-based, neurobiological reading disorder. It impairs a person's ability to read, and people with dyslexia read well below their expected reading level despite having normal intelligence. Dyslexia can be inherited, and scientists have identified a number of genes that may be implicated in its development.

When my youngest child, Warren, was about six years old, I discovered that he could not read. He had formed a habit of memorizing the words on the page but could not sound out words on his own. Given what I had endured as a child, I knew my approach to his learning issues would be different from what I had experienced. By the time Warren turned eight years old, his behavior in school had deteriorated significantly. Unable to understand and keep up with the classwork, he grew bored and became the class clown. He was enrolled in a Baltimore City public school, and I asked the school administrators to have him tested for learning issues. But the administrators were reluctant to do anything. They didn't see a boy struggling to read and find his place in the classroom.

Desperate, I did the only thing I knew at the time. I threatened to sue the school system. It was their responsibility to educate him, and they were failing. When Warren was finally tested and found to be dyslexic, he was sent to the Kennedy Krieger School, which operates education programs for children with a range of special needs. But he was kept in that program for only a year before he was transferred back to the public school system. He wasn't ready to return to a traditional classroom setting, and his progress lapsed again.

As a young mother, I didn't yet know enough to continue fighting for him to remain in the specialized program, and I didn't have the money to pay for a specialized private school like the Odyssey School or Jemicy School. For the next few years, Warren was transferred from one learning program to another, including some with small class sizes. Yet his learning problems continued, and his classroom behavior did not improve.

I hired a private tutor, who worked with small groups of children. But even in a setting outside a classroom, Warren still managed to be disruptive. His behavior was so bad, the teacher asked me not to send him back. With Warren there, she was unable to teach any of the other students. Frustrated, I enrolled him in a private school when he was about twelve years old, where he remained until he graduated high school.

Warren's troubles were not unique. About 15 percent of Americans have dyslexia, and while parents and communities can be great advocates for children with learning disabilities, the help that a child receives often comes down to the parents' financial resources.[1] Those who cannot afford a private education rely on public schools with limited resources. Many dyslexics who don't get help grow into adulthood never meeting their full potential.

•

Research has demonstrated that early identification and intervention are important factors in managing dyslexia and educating affected students. Yet parents, teachers, and students from across the state testified in 2008 that public schools in Maryland did not adequately address learning issues and dyslexia. I was disappointed that so many years after I had struggled to get the proper education for my son, families continued to struggle to receive educational activities and services appropriate for their learning-disabled children.

In 2015, after I was elected to the Senate, I cosponsored a bill to create the Task Force to Study the Implementation of a Dyslexia Education Program.[2] Senator Craig Zucker, who also had learning problems as a child, was the bill's primary sponsor. In addition to looking at then current practices for identifying and treating dyslexia in students in

Maryland public schools and in other states, the group was tasked with determining the appropriate structure to establish a dyslexia education program and developing a pilot program to implement the task force's recommendations in a limited geographical area. That bill was vetoed by the governor.

Regardless, the Task Force to Study the Implementation of a Dyslexia Education Program was formed under a similar bill. The task force noted in its December 2016 report that dyslexia is not acknowledged or identified as a condition of specific learning disability in Maryland public schools, even though it was included as a condition of "specific learning disability" in the Individuals with Disabilities Education Act.[3] This was particularly concerning because researchers have identified specific instructional methods and strategies that improve the reading skills in children with dyslexia.

Through public testimony and survey responses, Marylanders told the task force that Maryland school personnel were not consistent in acknowledging dyslexia as an educational condition. Rather, they saw it as a medical diagnosis or contended that identification of dyslexia was not required by special education law. Some school personnel also told parents that a reading disorder either cannot be detected until the child is in the third grade and exhibits a two-year gap in reading skills or that there is no way to test for dyslexia before a child learns to read. These gaps in knowledge about dyslexia and instructional approaches to help struggling readers needed to be addressed.

How could we address these shortfalls? The task force recommended six approaches to implement a dyslexia education program and to improve reading instruction for all students. Among the recommendations was the goal to recognize dyslexia as a condition of specific learning disability in all Maryland public schools, implement universal screening for all students starting as early as kindergarten, and develop a multitiered system of supports for struggling readers as well as a structured literacy approach for reading instruction for struggling readers and for all beginning readers in kindergarten through grade three. The task force also recommended changing the curricula and instructional strategies that tertiary institutions use for teacher training programs and implementing a Pilot Dyslexia Education Program that would serve as a model instructional system for effective reading instruction for all students.

Three years later, I cosponsored legislation to establish a screening program. The bill won approval, and the program was implemented at the start of the 2020–2021 school year. Each local school board must screen students to identify whether they are at risk for reading difficulties. Any student found to be at risk of reading difficulties must receive supplemental reading instruction. The bill also called for the Maryland State Department of Education to develop and update resources for local school boards every four years and provide technical support to local boards allowing them to provide training opportunities annually. Finally, I felt that what I had fought for on behalf of Warren was in place for other children.

That piece of legislation was of such significance for the students and parents who needed specialized instruction for reading difficulties that it earned me a Friend of Dyslexia Award from Decoding Dyslexia Maryland in 2020. The award itself notes my inspiration and advocacy for dyslexic youths. It's an honor I never could have imagined as a child struggling with reading or as a parent of a child with the same difficulties.

•

Studies show that educational equity goes hand in hand with health equity. Literacy is fundamental to academic success, and access to educational opportunities is one of the social conditions that has a profound impact on our health. Access to educational opportunities is also among the conditions the World Health Organization (WHO) classifies as the social determinants of health—the conditions in which people are born, grow, live, work, and age. I usually add another: the place where people die. And we can also argue that police brutality is a social determinant of health. These social determinants can include anything from safe housing to access to educational and economic opportunities, the quality of education, access to transportation and technologies, and socioeconomic conditions like poverty. Physical determinants include access to green spaces in the natural environment, exposure to toxic substances, accessibility of buildings and other physical structures, and design of housing and other structures.

Public health advocates tend to look at three areas where education and health intersect. First, health is necessary for education. A hungry child won't do well in school. Second, health education is part of the school curriculum, and in some jurisdictions, public health interventions occur in schools. Physical education is the third area.

There's another area of health that's closely tied to learning disabilities. A strong correlation exists between learning disabilities and substance abuse. Among teenagers, for example, researchers believe learning disabilities may lead to behaviors that overlap with substance abuse. The risk factors for the two are the same: lower self-esteem, difficulty with academics, feelings of loneliness, depression, and the desire to be accepted by their peers.[4] Diagnosing learning disabilities early is important. Moreover, dyslexia is rarely diagnosed alone. Researchers point to another comorbidity that dyslexia and substance use disorders share. Attention-deficit/hyperactivity disorder (ADHD) is the most frequent psychiatric disorder associated with dyslexia. Children with both dyslexia and ADHD are at an increased risk for substance abuse if they do not receive appropriate interventions.

This is the scenario I lived through with my son. Warren's learning disability is compounded by mental health issues and drug addiction, and even now as an adult, the problems that emerged in his childhood continue.

•

One afternoon, as I gave remarks before a group at the Loews Annapolis Hotel (now the Graduate Annapolis) in support of a bill championed by addiction counselors, I heard myself say, "I am the mother of an addict, and I have been through hell." The group had asked me to sponsor legislation to provide more funding for addiction counselors.

Until that point, I had not spoken publicly about my youngest son's addiction. Instead, I had heeded the counsel of other legislators who said that as a new legislator, I should not talk about it publicly. But I always believed in being forthcoming to get ahead of potentially damaging news before a challenger running against me brought it up.

I had not planned to discuss Warren's long battle with addiction, which emerged in his teen years and has continued through bouts of treatment and relapse throughout his adult years. But it felt important to talk about addiction, not only as a nurse and legislator but also to make it clear how deeply I understood the counselors' work and the type of issues they encountered. Drug addiction was a significant problem in the Baltimore City neighborhoods I represented. As I talked about the bill and my own experience as the mother of an addict, I felt as if I had stepped outside myself and heard my first public admission about the depth of pain that addiction brings to a family. Dealing with addiction is not easy for anyone involved. Not the individual suffering with the substance use disorder, nor the family members attempting to see the individual through various treatment programs.

"So from that perspective, I can understand the need for this piece of legislation," I said.

When I finished speaking, everyone in the room stood up to applaud. From there on out, each time I spoke about my son's addiction I had a line of people wanting to talk to me about their experiences— good and bad—and to thank me for speaking about an issue many of them were dealing with privately and some publicly.

The bill itself related to qualification and certification of certain categories of counselors who provided alcohol and drug counseling. I would go on to sponsor and cosponsor several pieces of legislation that dealt with alcohol and drug abuse treatment for the incarcerated and continued counseling support after they were released, as well as legislation that provided treatment for infants exposed to methamphetamine. One major bill, sponsored by Delegate Dan Morhaim, created the Maryland Governor's Task Force on Substance Abuse. I cosponsored the bill alongside Morhaim, who was also a medical doctor. The task force, led by Lieutenant Governor Kathleen Kennedy Townsend, developed a report that covered treatment programs and assessed what length of treatment was adequate.

Could we have done more? Absolutely. I knew that supporting former inmates through counseling for a year was ideal, but three months of support was all we could get for the legislation to pass. While the treatment program was good, our neighborhoods needed more comprehensive legislation to tackle such a pervasive problem that was plaguing the inner-city Black communities. Not until late in the 2010s did more legislators, health professionals, and counselors begin talking more broadly about opiate addiction; then the disparities around treatment in the Baltimore neighborhoods became more apparent to those outside our communities. In the Black communities, we had been talking about addiction and treatment for a long time, with little help. While predominantly Black young people died from addiction in large numbers in the city, legislators and the administration did not pursue comprehensive legislation to provide the necessary funding to explore programs that could make a difference. Treatment cannot exist in a vacuum: the high addiction rate, in some cases, is compounded by concentrated poverty and lack of jobs.

Another far-reaching piece of legislation created the Task Force on the Needs of Persons with Co-occurring Mental Health and Substance Use Disorders. The task force was meant to bring the substance abuse and mental health experts together to study the relationship between substance abuse and mental illness. How could we treat the whole person rather than one disorder at a time? This legislation also marked the first time the term "co-occurring disorders" was used in the General Assembly.

At that time in Maryland, the state had three programs serving youth, young adults, and homeless people with co-occurring disorders. The programs provided outpatient services and outreach to Native American and Hispanic community groups, developed transitional programs for adolescents and young adults with co-occurring substance abuse and mental disorders, and provided comprehensive clinical services and rental assistance.

Even so, a survey of licensed mental health providers by the Maryland Mental Health Coalition's Joint Workgroup on Co-occurring Disorders found that nearly 78 percent of respondents said people living in their area did not know what services were available for individuals with co-occurring disorders or how to access them. Another 58 percent said the current addiction treatment delivery system under HealthChoice (the state of Maryland's managed care program, or Medicaid) was not effective for people receiving the services, and nearly 64 percent said the current mental health delivery system was not effective for patients.

The reality of Warren's mental illness and substance use disorder meant not knowing which came first. Did his initial drug use stem from his first attempts to self-medicate? Or was his bipolar illness a result of his drug use? At the time that I introduced the legislation, the Report to Congress on the Prevention and Treatment of Co-occurring Substance Abuse Disorders and Mental Disorders estimated seven to ten million people in the United States had an alcohol or drug use problem and at least one mental disorder. The report, released in 2002 by the US Department of Health and Human Services' Substance Abuse and Mental Health Services Administration (SAMSHA), found that if one disorder is untreated, both disorders will worsen and can cause additional problems.[5] They should be treated simultaneously. Much later, SAMSHA invited me to a daylong conference on substance abuse and co-occurring disorders, and I was happy to see they were training providers on treating the whole person.

After the legislation had passed, I attended the Mental Health Association of Maryland's Mental Health Conference in Baltimore, where one of the presenters, a young man, confirmed the difficulty of inadequate treatment. "I wanted to die more than I wanted to live until I found a doctor willing to deal with my mental illness and substance abuse at the same time," the young man said. "Now I have a purpose.

I want to live more than I want to die." I heard similar testimony at the annual Black Mental Health Alliance for Education and Consultation Conference. That statement has stayed with me all these many years.

●

The kind of team approach to treat mental illness and substance abuse at the same time is exactly the type of approach that works for sickle cell disease, a severe hereditary form of anemia in which a mutated form of hemoglobin distorts the red blood cells into a crescent shape at low oxygen levels. Over the years, I found it hard to get funding for legislation related to sickle cell disease largely because of who it primarily affects. Sickle cell disease is particularly common among people whose ancestors are from sub-Saharan Africa and is estimated to occur among about 1 in every 365 Black Americans and 1 in every 16,300 Hispanic American births. Overall, about 1 in 13 Black babies is born with sickle cell trait in the United States.[6]

Sickle cell disease is a major, and costly, public health concern. Studies show that Americans with sickle cell disease have less access to comprehensive team care than people with other genetic disorders, such as hemophilia and cystic fibrosis. These crescent-shaped cells die early, which causes the patient to experience a constant shortage of red blood cells. When the cells travel through small blood vessels, they get stuck and clog the blood flow, causing pain and other serious problems such as infection and acute chest syndrome. The disease can also lead to strokes.

In my own work as a nurse, I had heard from sickle cell patients that their treatment, especially in a predominantly Black city like Baltimore, was often delayed. Patients in crisis generally showed up in the emergency room clutching an arm or any part of their body where the blood cells had clumped. Because drug addicts seeking pain medicine sometimes acted similarly, hospital staff tended to dismiss the sickle cell patient in crisis as a drug-seeking addict, relegating the patient to the back of the room where they would writhe in pain. That long wait for treatment often meant the sickle cell patient would need a blood transfusion to address the anemia, and in some cases, they would suffer organ damage because their clumped blood cells weren't getting necessary oxygen.

In 2007, I became involved in an effort to address the racial disparities in sickle cell treatment. At that time, in Maryland alone, about 1 in 400 African Americans had sickle cell disease, and 1 in 10 were carriers. African Americans then composed almost 30 percent of Maryland's population, and consistent with the distribution of the African Americans across the state, most sickle cell patients lived in the two major urban areas—the Baltimore metro area and Prince George's County.[7]

The Department of Health's 2006 Legislative Report assessed sickle cell disease management and the cost of care across the state.[8] According to the report, *The Hospital Discharge Database of the Maryland Health Care Commission*—which includes data covering all hospital admissions for sickle cell disease—between 2000 and 2005, there were 13,724 hospital admissions for adults with sickle cell disease. The average length of stay was 4.94 days, and the total cost of care was $97 million. About 26 percent of the admissions were covered by private insurance, 44 percent were covered by Medicaid, and 25 percent were covered by Medicare.[9]

While the data didn't distinguish between patients who were admitted to the hospital multiple times within a given year, it underscored that patients with sickle cell disease did not have a comprehensive system to manage their disease. And studies have long shown that comprehensive care is more cost effective than episodic care. Patients who have access to a comprehensive care clinic have fewer emergency room visits, require fewer hospital admissions, and, if they are hospitalized, stay in the hospital for a shorter period. All these factors lead to lower annual costs per patient.

The report recommended a series of steps to improve the quality of health care and health care delivery for adult patients with sickle cell disease, including (a) establishing a statewide steering committee to ensure that services for adults with the disease and their families were developed in such a way that they effectively serve the community, and (b) further developing the Sickle Cell Center for Adults at Johns Hopkins, the only comprehensive sickle cell disease treatment center in the state. The report recommended developing the treatment center as a day infusion center, which had been shown to lower costs and lead to better care. Studies demonstrated that day centers decreased hospital admissions by 43 percent and decreased the length of a hospital stay by 49 percent.[10] The report also promoted the use of standardized treatment guidelines and emergency room protocols, and an ongoing educational program for providers.

Implementing the recommendations was, of course, costly. Estimates of the funding needed to improve the quality of health care and reduce mortality rates for adults with sickle cell disease came in at about $2.2 million in the first year, and approximately $1.9 million annually after the start-up year.

One afternoon while I was on the Johns Hopkins University campus for an engagement, Larry Gourdine, my escort for the afternoon, invited me to attend a diversity committee meeting with medical staff. The doctors, nurses, and researchers in attendance discussed the challenges for sickle cell patients who arrived at the emergency room in crisis but sometimes waited for long periods before being treated. Knowing the potential for long-term damage to the internal organs of sickle cell patients in crisis, I was disturbed by what I was hearing. I told the group that I would put in legislation to address some of the issues. The first sickle cell bill I sponsored didn't pass. But the simple act of putting forth legislation spurred action.

Dr. Myron Weisfeldt of Johns Hopkins, who oversaw thirteen medical departments, and his colleague Dr. Sophie Lanzkrom joined forces with two managed care organizations, Priority Partners and Amerigroup, to create Maryland's first infusion center at Johns Hopkins dedicated to the treatment of sickle cell disease. The simple reality was that many of the patients Johns Hopkins treated on a regular basis were on Medicaid, and treating the patients early also meant lower overall costs for the hospital. When the center opened, it didn't operate around the clock, but over the years, the operating hours have expanded. Such centers should be in more communities, including Prince George's County, which has a high number of Black residents with sickle cell disease.

In 2007, I sponsored legislation that created a Statewide Steering Committee on Services for Adults with Sickle Cell Disease.[11] Getting the legislation passed enlightened me to a few things. Not all of my colleagues, especially those who lived in and represented districts with few African Americans, understood the gravity of sickle cell disease or even what it was. I took diagrams with me to meetings so I could show the members of various committees how a blood cell that is shaped like a sickle affects the whole body, why a person in crisis needs immediate intervention, and how sickle cell disease causes strokes and affects the lungs, kidneys, heart, liver, spleen, bones, eyes. I explained why patients with sickle cell disease often die young. I also started a Sickle Cell Day in the General Assembly, bringing constituents from across the state to talk to legislators and to educate them on sickle cell disease and the issues the patients confront.

The bill passed, establishing a steering committee that was required to build institution and community partnerships, as well as a statewide network of stakeholders who care for individuals with sickle cell disease; and to educate sickle cell disease patients, the public, and health care providers about options in Maryland to manage the disease. In addition, the committee was charged with seeking grant funding to develop and establish a case management system and day infusion center for adults with the disease. These centers have proven effective at reducing hospital admissions.

The committee issued a set of recommendations, including developing a statewide patient registry to facilitate counseling. The committee wanted to ensure that patients with the sickle cell trait knew ahead of time the potential that their offspring would have sickle cell disease. The registry also facilitated continuity of care across health care systems and providers, shifting resources toward comprehensive specialty care and preventive care models such as regional infusion centers, using the range of services provided by the Sickle Cell Infusion Center at Johns Hopkins as a model to be implemented in other parts of Maryland, and developing a standard protocol for sickle cell disease treatment in hospital emergency rooms and other urgent care settings.

While the legislation passed with $250,000 in funding for the work of the steering committee, the administration removed the funding after our first meeting. Consequently, the committee was without funding from May 2009 to July 2019 and did not meet. Recognizing the continued need for comprehensive treatment programs, in 2019, I sponsored another piece of legislation to reestablish the steering committee, hire additional staff, and increase the number of sickle cell disease infusion centers in Maryland.

The legislation passed and was signed into law, with an effective date of October 2019, a few months before the United States was confronted with the COVID-19 pandemic, highlighting with heartbreaking clarity how much death and disease could have been avoided if policymakers had been more aggressive in addressing the root causes of health disparities experienced by minority populations.

CHAPTER 13

Maternal and Infant Mortality

On a January morning in 2018, as Maryland delegates were gathering in Annapolis to begin the new legislative session, news broke that tennis icon Serena Williams was publicly discussing her potentially fatal childbirth experience for the first time.[1] Serena, who had won the Australian Open in 2017 and later announced that she had been pregnant during the tournament, underwent an emergency C-section when the baby's heart rate fell during contractions. While the birth went smoothly, by the next day Serena began experiencing shortness of breath. Since she had a history of blood clots, she immediately suspected she was experiencing another. Besides, she had temporarily stopped taking her daily anticoagulant medication in preparation for the surgery, which increased the possibility of another pulmonary embolism.

Serena knew what to ask for. She requested a CT scan and a heparin drip—a blood thinner—but the medical staff initially brushed aside her concerns as typical post-pregnancy symptoms and confusion from the pain medicine. Serena insisted, and before long she got an ultrasound on her legs and a CT scan. The scan revealed that several small blood clots had settled in her lungs.

Serena developed a number of health complications over the next six days—a surgery to repair the C-section wound that opened up from the intense coughing caused by the embolism, discovery of a large hematoma in her abdomen, and another surgical procedure to prevent clots from traveling to her lungs. Serena credited her recovery to access to a hospital with state-of-the-art equipment and an incredible medical team.

Serena's essay lifted a curtain on a public health problem that has been festering for decades. If this childbirth health scare could happen to Serena Williams, one of the most influential American athletes of the last two decades, what of the other women without her platform, voice, and access?

Later that same year, Grammy-award-winning artist Beyoncé Knowles also publicly discussed the health scare surrounding the birth of her twins in 2017. Beyoncé was diagnosed with preeclampsia, a pregnancy complication characterized by high blood pressure, protein in the urine, and signs of damage to another organ system, such as the liver and kidneys. Preeclampsia usually begins after twenty weeks of pregnancy in women whose blood pressure had been normal. Each year, roughly 5% percent of pregnant women in the United States are diagnosed with preeclampsia.[2] If left untreated, preeclampsia can lead to serious—sometimes fatal—complications for a mother and her baby. In Beyoncé's case, she had been placed on bed rest for about a month before having an emergency C-section. Both her life and the twins' lives were in danger.

Both women's stories reflect the grim reality for many pregnant women, especially African American women. What we know from recent studies is that African American women are three to four times more likely to die during or after delivery than are white women—a rate the World Health Organization (WHO) says is comparable to that of women in Mexico and Uzbekistan, where a large percentage of the population lives in poverty. In Maryland, the rate of maternal deaths was 26 deaths per 100,000 births for the five-year period of 2011 to 2015, based on data from the state's maternal mortality review board.[3]

How maternal death is measured varies. The WHO defines maternal death as "the death of a woman while pregnant or within 42 days of termination of pregnancy, irrespective of the duration and site of the pregnancy, from any cause related to or aggravated by pregnancy or its management but not from accidental or incidental causes." The Centers for Disease Control and Prevention (CDC) considers a pregnancy-associated death to be "the death of a woman while pregnant or within one year or 365 days of pregnancy conclusion, irrespective of the duration and site of the pregnancy, regardless of the cause of death." The CDC also defines a pregnancy-related death as "the death of a woman while pregnant or within one year of conclusion of pregnancy, irrespective of the duration and site of the pregnancy, from any cause related to or aggravated by her pregnancy or its management, but not from accidental or incidental causes."[4]

Interestingly, Beyoncé's and Serena's stories show that disparities in health care extend to Black women who are wealthy, are educated, and have access to best-in-class care.

Shalon Irving, an epidemiologist at the CDC, was not as lucky as Serena and Beyoncé. Shalon had spent her career focused on trying to understand how structural inequality, trauma, and violence contributed to poor health outcomes. She worked to uncover and eliminate inequity by focusing her research on how childhood experiences affect health at a later time.

Shalon knew she was at a greater risk during her pregnancy due to a clotting disorder and a history of high blood pressure. Like Serena and Beyoncé, she had access to quality health care. After delivering her daughter via C-section, her recovery was progressing well enough that her doctors allowed her to leave the hospital after two nights. Not long after she got home, her condition quickly deteriorated. Shalon visited her primary care providers several times, getting treatment for a hematoma—blood trapped under layers of healing skin—that developed at her incision, as well as for rising blood pressure, headaches, blurred vision, swollen legs, and rapid weight gain. But Shalon's doctors told her that the symptoms were normal. Within hours of her last doctor's appointment and three weeks after giving birth, Shalon collapsed and died from complications of high blood pressure.

Shalon had several things that should have worked in her favor. She had two master's degrees, a PhD, robust health insurance, and a job with the preeminent public health agency in the United States. But Shalon was also a Black woman. The CDC, the very agency for which Shalon worked, has said Black women face significantly higher maternal mortality risk than white women, with Black mothers in the United States dying at three to four times the rate of white mothers. Between 2014 and 2017, the CDC's data show 41.7 deaths per 100,000 live births for non-Hispanic Black women versus 13.4 deaths per 100,000 live births for non-Hispanic white women. Across all races, the maternal mortality rate has been trending upward. Since the CDC implemented its Pregnancy Mortality Surveillance System, the number of reported pregnancy-related deaths in the United States rose from 7.2 deaths per 100,000 live births in 1987 to 17.3 deaths per 100,000 live births in 2017. What was the cause of these deaths? Cardiovascular conditions, infection or sepsis, cardiomyopathy, hemorrhage, embolism, hypertension, or anesthesia complications.[5]

These statistics were startling, and especially so since America is one of the wealthiest countries in the world. Health care access, education, and money are not the driving factors. Inequities are.

•

How were these national trends reflected in my own home state?

Since the 2000 legislative year, Maryland has had a Maternal Mortality Review Program in place. That program was established to identify maternal death cases, review medical records and other relevant data, determine preventability of death, develop recommendations for preventing maternal deaths, and disseminate findings and recommendations to policymakers, health care providers, health care facilities, and the public. Each year, the program issues an annual report. Since 2018, the annual report has included a section on racial disparity.

The maternal mortality rate in Maryland showed a similar trend as the national trend toward a large disparity between the maternal mortality rate among Black and white women. Although Maryland's maternal mortality rate had declined over the past decade and at the time was below the national average, the racial disparity had widened, and significant racial disparities in maternal death persisted. Between 2012 and 2016, the Black maternal mortality rate in Maryland was 3.7 times that of white women. The report also found that compared with the 2007–2011 period, the 2012–2016 white maternal mortality rate in Maryland decreased 34.6 percent, and the Black maternal mortality rate increased 20.5 percent. Causes of death included cardiovascular and noncardiovascular medical conditions, homicide, suicide, cardiomyopathy, cerebrovascular accident, hemorrhage, and overdose.

These statistics, as well as Serena's, Beyoncé's, and Shalon's stories and others like them, weighed heavily on me, especially since researchers have determined that most pregnancy-related deaths are preventable. Overall, cardiovascular conditions are the main cause of pregnancy-related death among women. When maternal mortality is assessed by race and ethnicity, however, there are differences in the leading causes of death. The CDC's assessment of racial and ethnic disparities in pregnancy-related deaths in the United States between 2007 and 2016 found that cardiomyopathy, pulmonary embolism, and high blood pressure were associated with a higher share of pregnancy-related deaths among Black women compared with white women. A larger percentage of pregnancy-related deaths among non-Hispanic American Indian/Alaska Native women was tied to hemorrhage and high blood pressure compared with white women. Among Asian and Pacific Islander women, hemorrhage, amniotic fluid embolism, and cerebrovascular accidents were associated with a higher share of pregnancy-related deaths compared with white women. Hemorrhage and hypertensive disorders were associated with a higher share of pregnancy-related deaths among Hispanic women versus white women.

Importantly, the study noted that thirteen state maternal mortality review committees reported that 60 percent of pregnancy-related deaths were preventable.

Reducing disparities in pregnancy-related mortality requires a few key steps to address the multiple underlying factors. First is a strong data collection and analysis program as well as a robust set of recommendations and an action plan to reduce the disparities in pregnancy-related mortality. So at the start of the 2019 session, I proposed two pieces of legislation to address this pressing issue.

In the first, each county would be required to have a multidisciplinary and multiagency maternal mortality review team to prevent maternal deaths. The legislation supported the work of the statewide Maternal Mortality Review Program by creating mechanisms for local health offices to assemble a more focused, regionally responsive review team.

The second piece of legislation strengthened the state's maternal mortality review efforts by requiring the Maternal Mortality Review Program, in consultation with the Office of Minority Health and Health Disparities, to make recommendations to reduce any disparities in the maternal mortality rate, including recommendations related to social determinants of health.

•

As is the case with the maternal mortality rate, the infant mortality rate is highest among Black infants. While I was working to lower the maternal mortality rate in Maryland, I began looking at the infant mortality as well. Around that same time frame—the 2018 legislative year—the annual infant mortality in Maryland report indicated that the overall infant mortality rate in Maryland was 6.5 per 1,000 live births, a 3 percent decrease over 2015. Overall, 478 infants died in 2016, compared with 491 in 2015. It was particularly concerning that the infant mortality rate for non-Hispanic Black infants was higher than that of other racial groups—1.6 times the rate for all races/ethnicities and 2.4 times greater than the rate for non-Hispanic white infants. While we had little data on the infant mortality rate in rural areas of the state, 2016 data indicated that infant mortality rates in the Southern and Eastern Shore regions of the state were generally higher than the rates in other parts of the state. That year, the leading causes of death were disorders relating to short gestation and unspecified low birth weight, congenital abnormalities, maternal complications of pregnancy, sudden infant death syndrome, and complications of the placenta, cord, and membranes.[6]

To address the issue, it was important to understand all the underlying causes and seek possible steps to address early deaths in infants. That year, I sponsored legislation requiring a study of the mortality rates of African American infants and infants in rural areas. The proposed study would examine the factors affecting the mortality of African American infants and infants in rural areas in the United States and in Maryland and research programs intended to reduce the infant mortality rate. Researchers would also recommend methods to reduce the mortality rate of African American infants and infants in rural areas, ways to use pregnancy navigators or community health workers to assist pregnant women with the goal of reducing the infant mortality rate, steps to establish a permanent task force or work group for lowering rates of disparity with respect to infant mortality, and methods to reduce the costs associated with low-birth-weight infants and with infant mortality.

It was devastating to see little improvement between 2011, when Maryland published its last major plan to address infant mortality, and 2019, when the Maryland Health Care Commission published its *Study of Mortality Rates of African American Infants and Infants in Rural Areas.* That study originated from legislation I passed in 2017 requiring the Maryland Health Care Commission to study the mortality rates in that age group.

Based on the study, the numbers didn't improve despite changes in health care access, including expanded health insurance coverage under the ACA. The 2011 Plan for Reducing Infant Mortality in Maryland had a goal of reducing the infant mortality rate to 6.5 of every 1,000 live births by 2012. In 2017, however, the infant mortality rate remained the same, and researchers continued to see significant disparity in outcomes between Black and white infants. Among rural infants the mortality rate got worse, indicating that geography was also a factor that legislators, the administration, and health practitioners needed to consider. Among other issues, lack of adequate transportation in rural areas prevented mothers from getting prenatal care, leading to low-birth-weight babies with less than a fighting chance to survive.

The Health Care Commission made a number of recommendations, including improving existing processes to coordinate care, implementing rigorous implicit racial bias training in relevant health care providers' education and clinical practices, and improving continuity of care with, for example, the use of pregnancy navigators or community health workers to assist pregnant women with the goal of reducing the infant mortality rate.

What stays with me is that 68 percent of infant deaths occurred in the neonatal period or the first month of life, most likely due to factors related to the pregnancy itself and delivery. Black infants were four times more likely to die from low birth weight, twice as likely to die from congenital abnormalities, two and a half times more likely to die from sudden infant death syndrome, and thirteen times more likely to die from maternal complications of pregnancy.

The latter statistic is a strong indication of the persistent disparities in maternal mortality between Black and white women in Maryland. Fixing that persistent disparity in the mortality rates means addressing the impact of racism and bias, implementing strong implicit racial bias training for health care providers, and improving coordination of care and referring patients for mental health and substance use disorder treatment programs.

CHAPTER 14

Beyond Health Care

Social Determinants of Health

When I was running Nathan's Networks and actively visiting clients' homes between 1989 and 2015, I often saw empty refrigerators. Many families were struggling to survive. Sometimes I went to the supermarket and paid out of my own pocket or went to food pantries for the families. I told clients with transportation where the food pantries were located, even though food that's available at the pantries can be high in sodium and sugar—both harmful to already sick and vulnerable populations. Many of the clients I served were already suffering from high blood pressure and on renal dialysis.

While income and inadequate access to health care do not explain all health disparities, most disparities are rooted in unequal access to resources and opportunities. As I saw with Stella, those with higher education or income levels tend to have more access to and control over resources and opportunities.

How money, power, and resources at the global, national, and local levels are distributed often impacts social determinants and in turn is largely responsible for health inequities, or the unfair and avoidable differences in health status among different racial and socioeconomic groups across the United States. In Baltimore, for example, the health disparities sprout directly from the long history of inequality and systemic racism in housing, education, and policing that dates back to the written and unwritten policies that emerged during the recovery from the Great Depression.

In 2008, the World Health Organization's Commission on Social Determinants of Health published a report, *Closing the Gap in a Generation*.[1] The report outlined three recommendations to close the health gap by addressing social determinants of health:

- Improve daily living conditions, specifically the well-being of girls and women and the circumstances in which children are born. This approach put a large focus on early childhood development and education for girls and boys, as well as improving living and working conditions.
- Address inequities in how power, money, and resources are distributed.
- Measure and assess health inequity within countries and globally.

Establishing policies that impact social and economic conditions can make a dent in improving health for a large number of people. What I saw as a nurse and as the operator of two health care businesses told me that Maryland hadn't addressed the social factors that contributed to health equity. Too many of Maryland's residents were still falling behind in many areas. For example, early childhood development, including a child's fluency in letters and numbers, greatly affects the person's lifelong development. That's one of the reasons I worked over the years to establish educational programs, including programs that addressed dyslexia and learning problems. Education is just one factor that contributes to the persistence of unfair and unavoidable differences in health status among various communities across Maryland and America.

In the spring of 2015, the world saw anger about the persistent inequities play out in real time as protests about the death of a twenty-five-year-old African American man, Freddie Gray, spread across Baltimore. Gray had tried to run away when he saw the police, but they chased the young man and arrested him. A video recorded by a bystander showed the police officers dragging Gray into a police van after he was handcuffed. Gray was then transported to the station in the back of the van without a seat belt, with his hands and feet shackled. During Gray's transportation he suffered a severe spinal injury from which he never recovered.

Gray's death set off violent, dayslong riots in the neighborhoods near his home. The riots began as peaceful protests of a broader national issue: police mistreatment of Black men. Tensions across the nation were already high following two high-profile police brutality cases from the previous summer. In August 2014, police officers had killed Michael Brown, an unarmed Black teenager, in Ferguson, Missouri, a suburb of St. Louis. Soon after Brown's killing, residents in Ferguson began protesting his unjust killing. Protests and riots soon spread across the country. Nearly a month before Brown was killed, police officers attempting to arrest Eric Garner in the New York City borough of Staten Island choked him to death. The unarmed Garner was accused by police officers of selling untaxed cigarettes.

With tensions already high, the peaceful protests in Baltimore following Gray's death quickly escalated into more violent protests. While some residents expressed their anger over Gray's death by burning cars and buildings, another segment of the Baltimore population pointed to the underlying frustration over the lack of economic opportunities and mobility in certain Baltimore communities, and how little city officials had done to tackle the systemic issues contributing to a cycle of poverty.

It is easy to understand how social and economic issues became part of the national conversation about police mistreatment of Black men. Around April 2015, the unemployment rate in Baltimore was 8.4 percent, well above the 5.5 percent unemployment rate for the nation as a whole. The Baltimore City Health Department's 2017 neighborhood profile for the Sandtown-Winchester/Harlem Park area—Gray's neighborhood—indicated that 20.7 percent of the population of residents sixteen years of age and older were unemployed versus 13.1 percent for Baltimore City as a whole. To put it in context, nearly 97 percent of Sandtown-Winchester/Harlem Park residents are African American versus 63 percent for Baltimore City. The report showed that 16 percent of residents in Gray's neighborhood had no health insurance, and 51 percent of the residents had an annual income below $25,000. Fifty percent of families with children under eighteen lived in poverty, and only 6 percent of residents twenty-five years of age and older had at least a college degree, compared with 29 percent for Baltimore City as a whole.[2]

Statistics on the social determinants were just as stark. The youth homicide mortality rate—the rate of death due to homicide per 100,000 youth under twenty-five years old—was 68 in Sandtown-Winchester/Harlem Park compared to 31 for Baltimore City overall. The number of lead paint violations per 10,000 households per year in the neighborhood was 34.1 compared to 9.8 for Baltimore City overall. Lead poisoning occurs when lead builds up in the body, and it is a known cause of serious health problems, including developmental delays and learning difficulties. Gray himself, and his two sisters, had damaging lead levels in their blood when they were children, which led to multiple educational, behavioral, and medical problems. His family filed a lawsuit in 2008 against the owner of a Sandtown-Winchester home the family rented for a four-year period.

As a nurse, I know that every one of these social conditions affect overall health. As a legislator, I was determined to find ways to limit their effect on Maryland's residents. In February 2015, a few weeks before Gray's death and the riots broke out, I had convened a group of community leaders and health professionals in Annapolis—including members of the governor's office, the business community, and the National Association for the Advancement of Colored People (NAACP)—to discuss the social determinants of health and figure out what we could do. We named the project the Social Determinants of Health Workgroup in the 44th District. For years, I had been working to address some of these social issues in bills dedicated to single issues, but I wanted to tackle the problem of social determinants in another way.

I was pushed to form the work group because day after day I drove through my district in Baltimore City and saw young men just standing on the street corners. They were likely unemployed and uninvolved in their communities in any way. I wanted to see what we could do to address the lack of opportunities for residents in the Forty-Fourth District. Not long after we held our first meeting in Annapolis and convened a few meetings in the community, Freddie Gray died at the hands of police and the city erupted in protests.

The very issues being discussed by the Social Determinants of Health Workgroup in the 44th District were laid bare in the aftermath of Gray's killing. In 2018, I sponsored and won passage of a bill to establish the task force for a seven-year pilot in Baltimore City to assess the social determinants of health.

The task force's goal was to identify and examine the negative social factors that were causing hardships for Baltimore City residents, many of which span several generations and are cyclical. I wanted a task force that would not only study the issue but also develop and implement solutions that would improve the social, material, economic, and physical conditions in which Maryland residents lived, worked, played, and worshiped. Within the task force, five subcommittees would address specific issues: civil unrest and social justice; education; health and human services; housing; and workforce development and jobs.

For education specifically, the key areas the subcommittee would address were low graduation rate; the lack of adequate schools, materials, and opportunities for students; and violence and its effect on a child's ability to learn. The housing subcommittee would address the condition of housing in low-income areas, including blight and neglected housing and the presence of lead, mold, and pests. The workforce development and jobs subcommittee would address chronic unemployment and underemployment, job training programs, and employment of returning residents. The health and human services subcommittee would assess and address high morbidity and premature mortality; low birth rates; high rates of certain diseases, including hepatitis C, HIV/AIDS, diabetes, high blood pressure, cardiovascular disease, and stroke; suicide; mental illness; infant mortality; drug and alcohol abuse; and poor nutrition. And the civil unrest and social justice subcommittee would address various crises that affect Baltimore's neighborhoods, such as high incarceration rates and finding work for returning residents, as well as voter registration.

There's no easy fix. Back in 1972 when I met Stella, she had delayed medical care because she did not have a job and could not afford to pay for the care she needed. That situation plays out every day in America. In Baltimore especially, the unemployment rate remains high, with Baltimore City's rate often trending above national levels. In 2019, for example, the state's annual unemployment rate was 3.8 percent for 2018 and 3.4 for 2019. As of December 2018 and 2019, for example, Baltimore City's unemployment rate was 5.5 and 4.9 percent, respectively, versus 3.7 and 3.4 percent for the United States as a whole.[3]

While there's no simple solution, training residents for sustainable careers, particularly in the expanding technology and telecommunications fields, is one effective approach. By 2026, demand for workers in cybersecurity is expected to grow 13 percent. With a greater use of cloud computing, collection and storage of vast amounts of data, and the need to secure all that information from unauthorized use and access, cybersecurity jobs are growing at a faster rate than all other occupations. Why shouldn't youths in Baltimore have a chance to work in this growing field?

In 2018, I joined Senator Barbara Robinson as a cosponsor on her bill establishing the Cyber Warrior Diversity Program at several tertiary institutions—Baltimore City Community College, Bowie State University, Coppin State University, Morgan State University, and the University of Maryland Eastern Shore—to train students in computer networking and cybersecurity. The legislation provided $2.5 million for the program annually. A year later, I put in a second bill that made some minor changes to the original bill in terms of the schools that would be involved and listed University of Maryland Baltimore County (UMBC) as the university that oversees the training of cybersecurity students. The goal is to increase the number of people from underrepresented groups who earn certifications that allow them to work in the cybersecurity field.[4]

In the weeks leading up to the passage of the bill, several young men who had already been certified to work in the cybersecurity field testified about how their new career made a drastic difference in their lives. One spoke of transitioning from a homeless youth to a man contributing to his community and buying computers for the schools in his neighborhood. These are the kind of stories that remind me exactly what I set out to do when I began my political career.

•

Another piece of legislation passed and signed into law that year (2015) implemented behavioral health training for police officers through a pilot program in Baltimore City and County. By addressing behaviors that often lead to violent confrontations with citizens who are mentally unstable or addicted, I anticipated that such a program would lower the amount of money the counties pay out to the families of citizens harmed or killed by police action, including excessive or deadly force and false arrest. In the Freddie Gray case, for example, Baltimore City paid Gray's family a $6.4 million civil settlement. In 2020, the city of Louisville in Kentucky agreed to pay $12 million to the family of Breonna Taylor—a young woman killed by police officers who barged into her home to serve a warrant—and institute several police reforms. Other high-profile cases had similarly large amounts: $1.5 million to the family of Michael Brown, the unarmed Black teenager killed by a police officer in Ferguson, Missouri; $5 million to the Chicago, Illinois, family of LaQuan McDonald; and $3 million to the mother of Philando Castile, a Black motorist killed by a suburban Minneapolis police officer. Separately, Castile's girlfriend, who was sitting in the car during the incident, was awarded $800,000. Closer to home, a jury hearing a civil suit brought by the family of Korryn Gaines against Baltimore County awarded the family $37 million. Gaines was killed in August 2016 in an armed standoff with county police, and her young son was injured. The $37 million award was subsequently significantly reduced by an appeals court, and the case remains in litigation.

The financial impact of police misconduct on cities and taxpayers is a tremendous burden. While multimillion-dollar settlements are often talked about, lesser-known settlements are often in the thousands of dollars range. These costs add up. That money could be better spent. Preventing the violent confrontations is, of course, preferable.

Training police extensively in behavioral health is one approach the legislation contemplated. But, ironically, in the wake of Freddie Gray's death and the protests that followed, the Baltimore City police department no longer had the resources to pursue the pilot and form the Behavioral Health Task Force. In addition, the police commissioner who supported the pilot on behavioral health training and who was willing to work on the pilot program was removed from office. Baltimore County, however, had the resources but claimed their existing programs were sufficient. Since Gray's death, several other African Americans have lost their lives at the hands of police, including Gaines and two mentally ill men who were killed while their families were trying to talk them down.

The legislation, however, remains on the books. While it has not been activated, I still have hope the pilot will be implemented.

Another piece that would have made this program work was creating a restoration or stabilization center, where mentally ill persons or those with an addiction disorder would be taken instead of being arrested and taken to jail. The city of San Antonio in Texas has a similar program that provides a location where the mentally ill and addicted can get psychiatric treatment, counseling, and rehabilitation instead of a stint in jail. The program has saved city taxpayers upward of $50 million.

But in Maryland, the cost of building such a center was prohibitive, so the bill was never drafted. Baltimore City, however, established a stabilization center. As a nurse I had a different take on how it should be set up and run. I wanted a nurse practitioner to run the clinic and set standing orders for when someone who was brought in that was mentally ill or addicted to drugs that would include medical care, a social worker, and a psychiatrist or psychologist for mental health treatment.

•

Addressing these social issues was not always easy. Some bills made it to the floor and passed. Others died in committee. I didn't think, for example, that compassionate release for elderly inmates suffering from arthritis, cancer, end-stage renal disease, or any number of terminal illnesses would meet with opposition. But that particular piece of legislation did. Opponents to bills like these preferred to continue funding confinement of elderly inmates rather than allow them to go home and live out the remainder of their days with their families, and die in peace. Time after time, I testified that these elderly inmates would not even be able to kill a roach if they saw one.

Because of my work on behalf of inmates over the years, I'd earned a reputation as someone who looked out for prisoners.

"Your name is written on the bathroom walls in all of the prisons," Sue, one of my legislative aides, once told me.

Among inmates, I had become known as someone who championed their medical rights, and as a result I got boxes and boxes of mail from prisoners describing the poor conditions and the lack of adequate treatment from the correctional medical services. Back in 1996, I sponsored my first piece of legislation that directly affected inmates. That legislation provided state funding for alcohol and drug abuse treatment for inmates in the hope that successful treatment would lower the risk of recidivism. In addition, to help reduce drug addiction and the rate of recidivism, then Secretary of Public Safety and Correctional Services, Bishop Robinson, provided funding that covered treatment for three additional months following a person's release from prison. In 1997, I sponsored another piece of legislation to create a task force to study HIV exposure in Maryland's correctional facilities. The goal of the legislation was to understand how many people were affected and the screening process when inmates were admitted to correctional facilities.

A separate bill that directly affected inmates required the Department of Public Safety and Correctional Services, in collaboration with the Department of Human Resources and the Department of Health and Mental Hygiene, to develop a process to refer inmates diagnosed with hepatitis C to the Department of Human Resources or the Department of Health and Mental Hygiene for enrollment in Medicaid or the Primary Adult Care program upon release. The inmates also received counseling on managing hepatitis C and reducing transmission.

Every so often, I received letters from inmates begging for help for some of the elderly prisoners. One that stays with me is a letter from a wheelchair-bound inmate in his nineties who was in severe pain and asking for help. His request moved me to reach out to the medical director to see to it that the man got medicine to relieve his pain, and it prompted me to draw up legislation requiring compassionate release for elderly patients like these. Before the bill could even be heard, I got a letter from another inmate telling me the ninety-year-old man had died. We had not met, but his death broke my heart.

I cherish an arrangement of artificial red roses sent by an inmate who appreciated my efforts to help him obtain the medical and mental health treatment he needed. This particular inmate had been considered "crazy." But after I read about the trials and tribulations and diseases he contracted while he was in prison, I had to advocate on his behalf. When he was finally being treated as a human being, he felt so relieved that he sent me the roses.

•

I can't count the number of times I thought a proposed bill would pass easily only to be surprised by the fight it took to get it through committee and to the floor. Some never made it to the floor. Some issues—like same-sex marriage, abortion rights, the right to die, and gun control—are understandably difficult issues that generate strong support on either side. But even an issue like the sale and use of pesticides known to be harmful to children failed.

In 2017 and 2018, I sponsored legislation to ban neonicotinoids, a class of insecticides chemically related to nicotine. Neonicotinoids operate in much the same way as nicotine does. They act on certain kinds of receptors in the nerve synapse. These insecticides are more toxic to invertebrates, like insects, than they are to mammals, birds, and other higher organisms. Neonicotinoid insecticides are especially popular in pest control because they are water soluble, which allows them to be applied to soil and be taken up by plants.

While neonicotinoids were initially thought to be nontoxic to many beneficial insects, including bees, more recent studies show potential toxicity to bees and other beneficial insects through low-level contamination of nectar and pollen. Further studies indicate these pesticides may be harmful to humans.

Though we had support for legislation banning neonicotinoids, the first bill in 2017 was withdrawn. At the time, the administration and the leadership were not ready to pass the legislation, in part because the governor was pushing back against it. A number of farmers who use those pesticides, as well as manufacturers and large home improvement retailers, also came out against the bill. But in 2018, I again submitted the bill and it passed and became law without the governor's signature. Environmentalists and bee keepers were so exhilarated, they lined up outside the chamber in beekeeping suits, applauding me on the win and presenting me with bottles of honey with the bill number on it.

In 2019, my last year in the Senate, I sponsored a bill prohibiting the use of chlorpyrifos in the state. The ban would include insecticides that contain chlorpyrifos or seeds treated with chlorpyrifos. Studies have confirmed that chlorpyrifos causes neurodevelopmental issues and cancer in children and the elderly and is the second most harmful pesticide for pollinators. Four years before I sponsored the bill, scientists at the Environmental Protection Agency (EPA) confirmed that chlorpyrifos could not be considered safe at any detectable level and recommended that the pesticide be banned. The Trump administration later reversed the EPA's decision.

Despite the scientific evidence, my bill didn't move forward to the Senate floor. I was disappointed but not defeated, and I vowed to propose the bill again. Although I retired before I could reintroduce the bill, I made sure that a colleague, Senator Lam, moved it forward, and in the 2020 session a new bill banning the pesticide passed, but it was vetoed by the governor. I have hope that future legislation banning the pesticide will become law. Our lives depend on our ability to limit exposure to known carcinogens like chlorpyrifos.

•

Over the years, I have learned that legislators and state and federal administrations have to tackle health disparities and social determinants with multiple initiatives. In 2017, I tried a different approach and put forth legislation to require a work group of state and nonstate agency representatives to apply the Health in All Policies (HiAP) framework to address disparities. Health in All Policies—a program headed by Stephen Thomas, who served as director for the University of Maryland School of Public Health's Maryland Center for Health Equity—addresses the social determinants of health that are the key drivers of health outcomes and health inequities.[5] The legislation requires the Center for Health Equity, in consultation with Maryland's Department of Health, to convene a work group to study and recommend laws and policies that will have a positive impact on the health of Maryland residents.

The work group was charged with examining and making recommendations on incorporating health considerations into decision-making, fostering collaboration among state and local governments, and developing laws and policies to improve health and reduce health inequities, as well as presenting recommendations on how those laws and policies are implemented. Among the factors the work group examined were access to safe and affordable housing; educational attainment; opportunities for employment; economic stability; inclusion, diversity, and equity in the workplace; barriers to career success and promotion in the workplace; access to transportation and mobility;

social justice; environmental factors; and public safety, including the impact of crime, citizen unrest, the criminal justice system, and governmental policies that affect individuals in prison or released from prison.

The work group made several recommendations, including establishing a Health in All Policies Council to develop a Maryland Health in All Policies Framework and implement a process for data sharing among state agencies. The work group also recommended developing a Health in All Policies Toolkit to help state agencies, legislators, and policy directors understand what Health in All Policies is and how to implement it into their operations. I hoped the work group would have developed examples of health policies unique to various departments that addressed how specific issues affect health. For example, the Department of Housing should have a health policy that speaks specifically to lead paint poisoning, rodents, and mold and addresses the many health issues that often plague children in public housing. The Department of Transportation's health policy should address the impact of emissions and air quality and asthma and COPD, while the Department of the Environment's health policy should look at the impact of brown fields and carcinogens on health. While these policy examples were not part of the report, I was pleased with the holistic approach to solving social determinants of health and addressing the external factors that can have a big impact on life expectancy and health.

CHAPTER 15

Lasting Legacy and Advocacy

My second campaign for the Senate in 2018 was the most brutal campaign of my thirty-year career as a politician. I first ran for the Senate seat in 2014 when redistricting of Baltimore County and Baltimore City placed me in the new Forty-Fourth District of Maryland. It was a hard decision to run against Senator Verna Jones, whom I liked and respected. The incumbent senator, however, had represented only 25 percent of the new district, while I had been the representative for more than 75 percent of the district. For that reason, I decided to run, and I won that seat.

But four years later, the Service Employees International Union (SEIU), one of Maryland's most powerful labor unions and a group that had previously supported me during my campaigns for the House, decided to support a challenger instead. The SEIU tends to champion health care, and while I was in the House I worked diligently and supported the union on various health care initiatives. In the midst of the campaign, I found myself looking back on photos of me standing among SEIU members at rallies and protests holding up signs. Losing the union's support stung.

In the end, I won, garnering more than 85 percent of the vote during the primary. And on January 9, 2019, I was sworn into the Senate for my second four-year term. That year, I was one of six lawmakers in the Maryland General Assembly of Caribbean descent. When I was elected to the House in 1994, I was the first Caribbean-born person to be elected to the General Assembly in its over 300-year history. I was proud of that and equally proud that for the first time, there were six Caribbean-born representatives serving in the Maryland General Assembly—two senators and four members in the House. We represented Trinidad and Tobago, Jamaica, Barbados, and the Dominican Republic. I took the opportunity to recognize the contributions people from the Caribbean islands have made to Maryland by sponsoring legislation proclaiming August as Caribbean Heritage Month in Maryland. The proclamation, which the governor issues each year, urges educational and cultural organizations to observe Caribbean Heritage Month with appropriate programs, ceremonies, and activities. We kicked off the first celebration in August 2019 in Silver Spring, Maryland, with a presentation by Dr. Franklin Knight, Jamaican-born Stulman Professor Emeritus of History at Johns Hopkins University, on the history of the Caribbean and a church service at St. Bartholomew's Episcopal Church.

The fall months leading up to the election and immediately after were difficult and exhilarating. Besides the campaign, I was inducted as a fellow of the American Academy of Nursing, one of the most prestigious awards given to people in my profession. I also received the 2018 Senator of the Year Award from the Maryland Black Caucus Foundation during its Annual Legislative Black Caucus Weekend festivities. I was especially proud of this award because I was one of the four founding members of the Black Caucus Weekend activities. Delegate Talmadge Branch, Delegate Salima Marriott, Senator Larry Young, and I modeled weekend activities after the Congressional Black Caucus annual event, which each of us always supported.

My body, though, wasn't keeping up with all I demanded it do. Weeks earlier, I had two cataract surgeries, and complications from one of the surgeries required emergency treatment. After the November election, I took a trip to Jamaica and Florida, but I became ill in Jamaica and could not enjoy my stay. I was later diagnosed with epiglottitis—an inflammation in the epiglottis, which can be deadly if not treated early.

I began the 2019 session already under the weather. I was so fever-ish, Sharon and Wayne drove down from Baltimore the night before the session was set to begin to help me get ready for the swearing-in ceremony. They brought with them Jamaican white rum and lime—the age-old Jamaican cure to lower fevers—and rubbed the mixture on my neck, chest, and back, then stayed overnight to watch over me. I made it through that day and through the session, fighting for the twenty-three pieces of legislation I had introduced, acutely aware that my body was weary. Still, I accomplished a lot, getting several bills passed and signed into law, including bills covering the treat-ment of hepatitis C and sickle cell anemia; the development of a cy-bersecurity training program; funding for a program requiring the Maternal Mortality Review Program to include data on racial dispari-ties; and funding for a bill to address learning disabilities and dys-lexia. But new health challenges emerged, and a long-standing con-dition with my spine reared up again, so strongly I needed a third surgery and months of physical therapy.

Those last months were marked by tremendous pain. Walking even a short distance took a lot out of me. I powered through, walking slowly and deliberately from the Senate building to the House of Delegates to talk to legislators about passing the hepatitis C bill, to beg for the vote to come up, and to ask the fiscal department to find additional funds so the bill could cover a greater number of hepatitis C patients on Medicaid.

Some days the pain was so bad, my staff drove me from one build-ing to another. I walked with a cane, stopping every five or so steps to allow the pain to ease. While I always stopped to greet the security per-sonnel and reception staff, what nobody knew then was that each stop to say hello was an opportunity for me to rest before taking an-other five steps.

I was too vain to use a motorized scooter or a roller walker. I didn't want to be pitied. Knowing I needed to let my body rest, I made the hard decision to retire. It was especially difficult because I still had three more years ahead on my term and more work I wanted to accomplish.

•

The first news of the novel coronavirus strain (COVID-19) came to me on a January morning, a few weeks after I had retired. I watched the early reports of the coronavirus spreading globally. When I first heard about COVID-19, it had not yet been diagnosed in the United States, but Wuhan, the city in China where the virus is thought to have first infected humans, had already locked down and limited movement in and out of the city in order to control the virus's spread. Another few weeks passed before the first COVID-19 case was diagnosed in the United States, followed by a gradual and then rapid spread to all fifty states and the District of Columbia. Pretty soon we were in the midst of a global pandemic, characterized by a range of responses across Asia, Europe, Africa, and the Americas.

All my life's work had taught me that communities of color and the underrepresented, marginalized communities would suffer most. Many of the preexisting health conditions that increased the risk of death from COVID-19 were the very conditions that research has shown disproportionately affect communities of color and poor communities. In addition, long-term neglect of health and racial disparities and the reduction of services in communities of color also increased the likelihood that these communities would fare the worst.

In fact, many African Americans hold jobs in industries that put them at greater risk: health care, including those working in a nonmedical capacity in the hospital setting, nursing home staff, and home health aides; retail service; and transportation. For many of these employees, remote work and social distancing were not options. Low pay, lack of medical insurance, and lack of paid sick leave compound the issues. By mid-March, it became clear that the racial and health inequities that had been evident all along would play out in the COVID-19 pandemic. Black and brown communities were disproportionately affected by the virus.

The COVID-19 pandemic's impact on Black and brown communities was the strongest evidence of the attention I had strived over the years to bring to racial and health inequities and prioritize these concerns in legislation. Had we implemented various recommendations to reduce disparities and provided full funding for these programs, we would be telling a different story about the burden of COVID-19. Legislative bodies across the country have never provided adequate funding for programs to help reduce racial disparities and the morbidity and mortality rate among marginalized groups: COVID-19 made this abundantly clear.

When I think back about how legislators fail to fully address a problem, particularly when the issue predominantly affects Black and brown communities, I think back to my legislative efforts to address sickle cell anemia. In 2007, my legislation to create a task force to address treatment of sickle cell anemia passed with a $250,000 fiscal note. A fiscal note is a written estimate of the costs, savings, and revenue gain or loss that may result from implementing a bill. A fiscal note doesn't guarantee funding, and in the case of a statewide budgetary shortfall, funding promised under a fiscal note can be taken away, which is exactly what happened with the sickle cell bill. At our first meeting, the governor removed the $250,000 funding, severely crippling the task force's work.

More often than not, I have found that legislation that primarily impacted the lives of Black people passed but did not get funding. That was the case with the Office of Minority Health and many other pieces of legislation.

As I watched the initial federal response to the pandemic, I thought of Dr. Martin Luther King Jr.'s words: "Of all the forms of inequality, injustice in health care is the most shocking and inhumane." This isn't the most popular of Dr. King's quotes, but it is the one that I lived by, and the message that underpinned the issues I fought to solve from the moment I set foot in Annapolis as a freshman delegate and throughout my entire career.

Though I had retired, I stepped back into a role I knew best. Perhaps I had not really left it behind after all. News of the devastating and disproportionate rate of deaths of African Americans was overwhelming. Even more disheartening was the tepid response. I wanted to see a more urgent national response that matched the state of emergency that Maryland and other states had already declared. And I wanted to see a broad, national collection of racial data to not only understand the scope of the pandemic in communities of color but to direct the needed resources to treat the virus, including broader testing, protective equipment, and proper access to treatment.

My hometowns of Baltimore City and County were hit hard, and I spent many evenings during the lockdown convening virtual meetings of nurses, doctors, public health officials, and various health care providers, together with the members of the Social Determinants of Health Task Force. The West Baltimore Initiative was led then by Christopher Gibbons, MD, who worked with Simmons Memorial Baptist Church to launch a community-based COVID-19 screening, testing, and counseling center in the West Baltimore neighborhood. These were the areas with the highest number of cases. We put the pieces together to ensure health care providers had access to resources, including personal protective equipment, to fight the virus and protect the community.

There are other projects that I remain involved in, such as the Task Force on Reconciliation and Equity, which was convened to examine the impact of institutional and structural racism across a wide cross section of areas including health, education, criminal justice, and faith-based initiatives and to suggest solutions and areas for improvement. The idea for the conversations on reconciliation came about following a meeting of my church's adult forum, which usually meets on Sunday mornings. One morning after a discussion on reconciliation, one member, Jack Lattimore, asked me to do something, and I followed up with the bill called Morgan State University Reconciliation and Equity, a Conversation on Race. That was the first state- and national-level task force of its kind in the United States. The task force, developed under Morgan State University's Institute for Urban Research, follows the model South Africa and other nations adopted to address the legacy of racism. The task force's report includes recommendations in the areas of health, criminal justice, and education. Some of the discussions on racism that I wanted to see occur between the Black, brown, and white members of the task force, however, didn't happen to the extent that I had hoped, largely because the pandemic prevented the task force from meeting in person and because it got off to a slow start. I had worked hard to get funding to finish the task force's work, including $25,000 that the House and Senate found. But the governor, who controls the funds, would not release them. That slowed our progress, and we didn't accomplish all that we set out to do, so the final report fell short of my expectations.

The legislation requires the task force to interview Marylanders in all twenty-three counties and Baltimore City on racism and its impact on their lives. Even though we could not meet in person, I worked with legislators across party lines to identify people who could speak on several issues affecting racism. In the end, we obtained and recorded interviews from residents representing over 50 percent of the counties. These virtual testimonies were recorded and compiled as an addendum to the final report sent to the Maryland General Assembly in January 2021. Collecting the data would not have been possible without the expertise of media personality Walter Kirkland. To my knowledge, due to the pandemic, the recommendations have not yet been addressed.

I remain involved with the Social Determinants of Health Task Force and the Health in All Policies Task Force, which submitted its recommendations to the Maryland General Assembly in January 2020. Again, due to the pandemic, we have not yet seen the outcome of the work of the task force.

•

On paper, I am retired, but in reality I am not. Even in 2020, 125 years after W. E. B. Du Bois and Booker T. Washington talked about the deficiencies in Black health care during and post slavery, the problems Stella faced—lack of access to quality health care and unemployment—still exist. For Stella and other unemployed persons, the problem is compounded by the fact that for most Americans, health insurance and health care is tied to their employment.

All these projects and all these stories lead to one thing that needs to change in America: the refusal to provide the necessary understanding of the economic impact of inadequate health care on Black and minority health. In 2011, researchers Dr. Thomas A. LaVeist, Dr. Darrell Gaskin, and Dr. Patrick Richard published a study on the costs—both direct health care costs and indirect costs such as loss of productivity—of racial health inequalities. The authors of the study, *Estimating the Economic Burden of Racial Health Inequalities in the United States*, conducted three sets of analysis.[1] The researchers assessed direct medical costs and indirect costs to estimate the potential cost savings of eliminating health disparities for racial/ethnic minorities and the productivity loss associated with health inequalities for racial/ethnic minorities. The group also assessed the costs of premature death.

The researchers found that for the 2003 to 2006 time frame, eliminating health disparities for minorities would have reduced direct medical care expenditures by about $230 billion. Indirect costs associated with illness and premature death would have dropped by more than $1 trillion for the same time period. (All figures are 2008 inflation-adjusted dollars.) The study clearly showed that addressing health disparities can be cost effective.

The report led to legislation authorizing Health Enterprise Zones (HEZs)—specific geographical areas targeted to received state resources to reduce health disparities, improve health outcomes, and reduce health costs and hospital admissions and readmissions. The legislation provided $4 million per year over the program's four-year term, as well as a range of incentives and resources for the HEZs, including grants and tax credits.

In 2016, three and a half years after the program was put in place, the Maryland Department of Health and the Community Health Resources Commission reported significant accomplishments, including opening or expanding twenty-two health care delivery sites and recruiting service providers to meet patient needs. Despite the successes, including saving the state more than $50 million, the HEZ program was discontinued. This is an ongoing problem in government. A new administration takes office and dismantles programs rather than build on successes. This was one such program where the successes should have been seen as the foundation for further development of the program.

Yet, twelve years after the authors published their study on the economic burdens of racial health inequalities, we still have a long way to go. Nearly forty-four years have passed since I first met Stella. Maryland has made significant strides in curing some of the issues that led to Stella presenting in the hospital with advanced cancer. The Affordable Care Act, implemented in 2010, makes affordable health insurance available to a broader segment of Americans and provides subsidies to Americans like Stella. These subsidies lower insurance costs for households with incomes between 100 percent and 400 percent of the federal poverty level. In some states, it also expands the Medicaid program to cover all adults with income below 138 percent of the federal poverty level.

The COVID-19 pandemic caused another wrinkle: Almost 10 million workers have lost access to the health insurance they received through their employer.[2] By the time the economy fully recovers from the shock of the pandemic, that number may be significantly higher. These estimates of the number of Americans without health insurance exposes the uncertainty that comes with health insurance provided solely via employment. Each economic crisis or employment setback increases the health and financial risks for families. Studies have shown us over the years that those most likely to suffer from this type of economic setback and loss of health insurance and health care are Black and brown communities, the very communities that are already greatly impacted by disparities in health care. One of my fears is that these crises will produce many more Stellas.

The solution is one that has been proposed time and time again. It is time to do away with employer-based health care plans and create a public health care system that provides coverage regardless of employment status or a family's financial situation. Several developed nations—England and Canada are great examples—have systems in place that provide a model of the type of coverage that the United States should consider. The long-term solution to this problem is a strong public option for insurance coverage. America's goal should be creating a public option that is the default insurance for most Americans.

Without a public health care system that is not tied to an individual's employment, I fear that each economic crisis like that created by the COVID-19 pandemic will produce many more people like Stella with a variety of ailments who need and can't afford early intervention to prevent needless death.

We are a long way from achieving equity. But I'm comforted by the work Maryland legislators are doing today to further the work I began many years ago. In the 2021 session, Delegate Joseline A. Pena-Melnyk introduced legislation in the House and Senator Mary L. Washington sponsored the companion bill in the Senate to create a commission to examine the health of Maryland residents and how factors such as affordable housing, education, and employment affect health outcomes. The commission would advise the state government on racial, ethnic, cultural, or socioeconomic disparities in health and set goals for health equity. The bill—the Shirley Nathan-Pulliam Health Equity Act of 2021—honors the work I've done over the years to shed light on racial disparities and their impact on health outcomes. Even this step forward is not without controversy. Late in the legislative process, after the proposed legislation had already passed out of committee to the floor, objections from Republican and some conservative Democrat lawmakers spurred changes to the bill, and all references to past and present racism were removed in favor of moving the bill forward without an extended fight. Over three decades earlier I faced a similar struggle to shed light on the impact of racism on health disparities. Even now, with the coronavirus pandemic exposing the breadth of systemic racism on disparities, the struggle remains.

For decades I spoke out, declaring that racism, which puts certain communities and individuals at a disadvantage, is a public health crisis. Others agree, including Dr. Patricia Newton, a renowned psychiatrist who died suddenly in 2021, who asked me to make sure the legislature cites racism as a public health crisis. I still say the same today. We have to be willing to see it as such and take bold steps toward righting these wrongs.

Trying to save and speak out for the Stellas of the world has been and remains an ongoing effort for me. I am forever moved by Dr. Martin Luther King Jr's statement: "Our lives begin to end the day we become silent about the things that matter."

I am not silent.

Not yet.

•

For the past twenty-eight years, the first thing I have seen upon waking is a lithograph called the *Wrapping of Cloth* by artist Gilbert Young. It has hung on my bedroom wall as a reminder of my three lives—my early years in Jamaica, my late teen years in England, and my adult years in the United States. The first woman in the painting is fully naked to the world. The second woman, partially clothed from the waist down, evolves from the shoulder of the first woman. The third woman, fully clothed, evolves from the hips of the second woman. This metamorphosis reminds me of nature and how a caterpillar evolves into a cocoon and then opens up into a beautiful butterfly.

Each stage represents me in different times of my life. The fact that the women's faces are not seen fully is telling. In the first stage, the woman's face is fully turned away, in the second her head is bent down and partially turned away, and in the final view her silhouette shows a confident woman looking toward the future.

The painting further reinforces to me that none of us are fully self-actualized. At all stages of life, we are yearning to accomplish something significant. I've measured my life by the belief that as long as I am living and breathing, I can do more, regardless of my age. The moment we stop learning is the moment we are ready to die. I want that to be my legacy for the generations to come—in Jamaica, in the Caribbean, and across the Americas, and specifically for young women and nurses. Living a life that matters is not about what you get from somebody but what you give. With all my years of working hard, giving back, and remembering that *can't* is not in my vocabulary, I believe strongly that in trying to improve the quality of life for all people, I have lived a life that mattered. All my life as mother, nurse, businesswoman, and legislator, I looked for ways to get around obstacles.

I think back to my childhood difficulties with learning, the way I looked at my disability as an obstacle, and how I learned, as a young adult, to manage the difficulties by approaching learning differently and taking my time. I didn't give up. I fought through the obstacles and accepted that I was not—just as I am not now—fully self-actualized but still yearning to learn. We grow. We change. We evolve. We find a way around the obstacles. All my life as a legislator I looked for ways around the obstacles. *Can't* was never in my vocabulary then. And it isn't now. I don't think of what I can't do. I think of what I can.

When I look back, it is comforting to see the results of that approach. My work has been recognized in various ways. I was honored by the American Public Health Association with a lifetime achievement award, named a Maryland Top 100 Woman three times, and named to the *Daily Record*'s Circle of Excellence. The Center for Health Equity at the University of Maryland College Park and the Maryland Department of Health established the annual Shirley Nathan-Pulliam Health Equity Lecture series. My alma mater, the University of Maryland School of Nursing, named me a visionary pioneer, established an endowment for a scholarship in my name, appointed me to the Board of Visitors, and honored me with the Dean's Medal for Distinguished Service. On May 18, 2023, I was conferred an Honorary Doctorate of Public Service at the university. I received the First Citizen's Award from the Maryland Senate, received an honorary doctorate in Humane Letters from Coppin State University, and witnessed the Maryland legislature name a bill after me, the Shirley Nathan-Pulliam Health

Equity Act of 2021. For my work in health disparities, I received two Congressional Honors, from Senator Ben Cardin of Maryland and Congresswoman Yvette Clarke of New York. The University of Maryland has built a student center at the School of Nursing that carries two engraved names at the top of the building for future nurses to see: my own—Nathan-Pulliam—and Esther McCready, a nurse who recruited Thurgood Marshall to sue the University of Maryland Baltimore nursing school to allow Black students.

Still, my work is not finished. I tried to make a difference and improve the quality of life for all people.

And I am still trying.

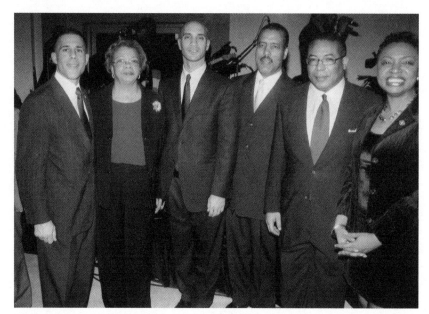

Left to right: Anthony Brown, lieutenant governor of Maryland; the author; Adrian Fenty, then mayor of Washington, DC; Gordon Shirley, then Jamaican ambassador to the United States (2004–2007); Tony Hilton, member of Jamaican Parliament; and Congresswoman Yvette Clark of New York honored by the Embassy of Jamaica in 2006 at the Reagan Center in Washington, DC

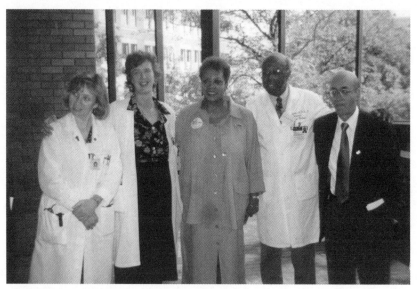

University of Maryland Greenbaum Cancer Center after signing breast cancer legislation, 1998

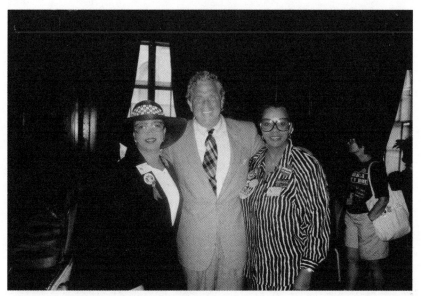

Left to right: Sandra Gray; Mike Miller, president of the Maryland Senate; and the author at the 1992 Democratic National Convention in New York City

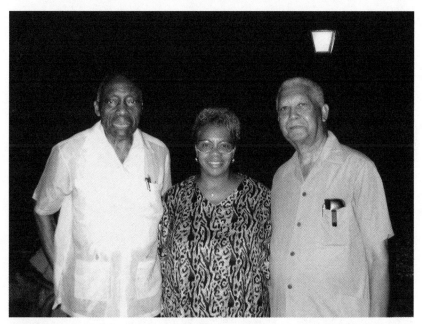

Left to right: Keith Johnson, then Jamaican ambassador to the United States (1981–1991); the author; and E. Leopold Edwards, O.D., at the author's home in Baltimore

Baltimore Ravens visit to Annapolis, Maryland (*left to right*): Brian Billick, the author, David and Art Modell, and Ozzie Newsome

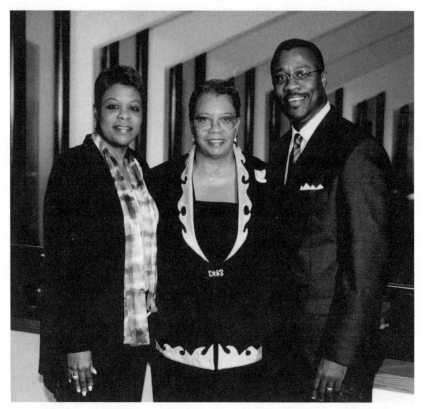

Left to right: Sharon J. Pulliam, the author, and Wayne A. Pulliam at Maryland's Top 100 Women awards ceremony (Shirley Nathan-Pulliam, awardee)

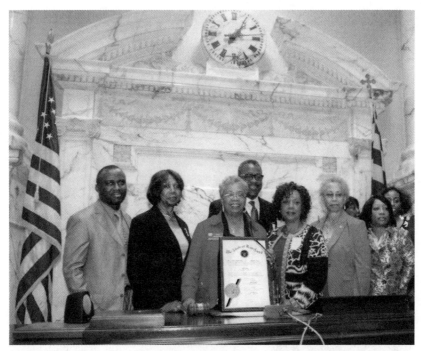

Swearing-in ceremony to the Maryland Senate, 2015, surrounded by family and friends

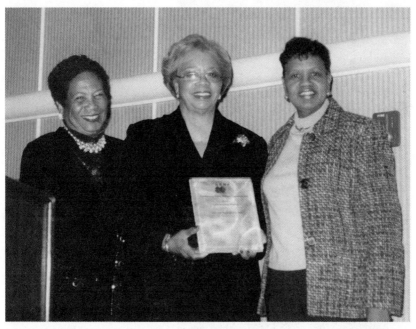

Left to right: Dr. Linda Bolton, the author, and Dr. Alicia George at the National Black Nurses Association Conference in Washington, DC

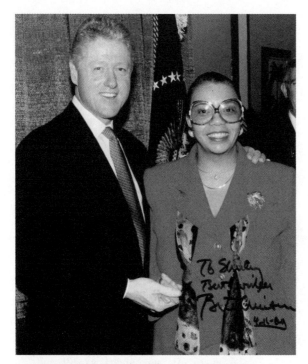

President Bill Clinton congratulates Delegate Shirley Nathan-Pulliam and the Maryland General Assembly after passage of Maryland gun control legislation (modeled after the Brady Bill), 1997

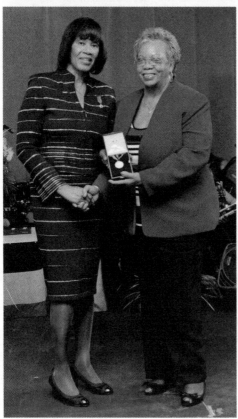

With the Most Honorable Portia Simpson-Miller, then prime minister of Jamaica, at the Prime Minister Appreciation Award ceremony in Kingston, Jamaica, 2014

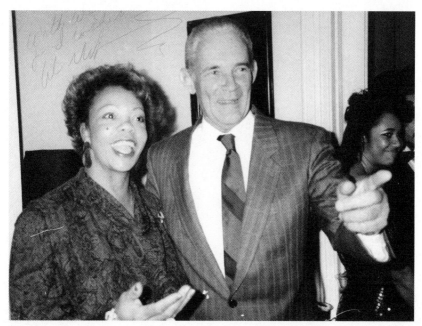

With the Most Honorable Michael Manley, former prime minister of Jamaica, in Silver Spring, Maryland, 1986

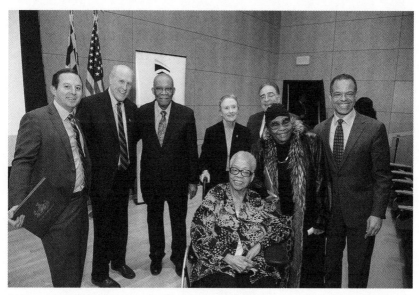

Left to right: Bill Ferguson, president of the Maryland Senate; Bruce Jarrell, MD, FACS, president of the University of Maryland, Baltimore; Professor Larry Gibson, University of Maryland School of Law; Jane Kirschling, PhD, then dean of the University of Maryland School of Nursing; Chancellor Jay Perman, MD, University System of Maryland; Barbara Robinson, former senator of Maryland; Malcome Augustine, president pro tempore, Maryland Senate; and the author at the honoring and naming of one of the buildings at the University of Maryland School of Nursing in 2023

Chapter 4. Learning the Modern American View of Race

1. *Census of Population and Housing, 1960*, Final Report Series PHC (1), Census Tracts, prepared by the Population Division in cooperation with the Housing Division, United States Census Bureau (Washington, DC, 1961), https://www.census.gov/library/publications/1961/dec/population-and-housing-phc-1.html.

2. *Census of Population and Housing, 1960.*

3. Antero Pietila, *Not in My Neighborhood* (Chicago: Ivan R. Dee, 2010).

4. Mary Seacole, *The Wonderful Adventures of Mrs. Seacole in Many Lands* (New York: Penguin Books, 2005).

5. Jean Marbella, "The Fire Both Times: Baltimore Riots After Martin Luther King's Death 50 Years Ago Left Scars That Remain," *Baltimore Sun*, March 28, 2018.

6. Pietila, *Not in My Neighborhood.*

Chapter 5. Becoming a Community Activist

1. W. E. B. Du Bois, *The Souls of Black Folk: Essays and Sketches* (Chicago: A.C. McClure, 1903).

2. Vanessa Northington Gamble and Deborah Stone, "Booker T Washington and Du Bois: Disparities, Research, and Action: The Historical Context," excerpted from "U.S. Policy on Health Inequities: The Interplay of Politics and Research," *Journal of Health Politics, Policy and Law* 31, no. 1 (February 2006): 93–122, 99–108, https://academic.udayton.edu/health/11Disparities/Disparities07.htm.

3. W. E. B. Du Bois, "The Health and Physique of the Negro American," *American Journal of Public Health* 93, no. 2 (February 2003): 272–76, https://doi.org/10.2105/ajph.93.2.272.

4. Du Bois, "The Health and Physique of the Negro American."

5. Gamble and Stone, "Booker T Washington and Du Bois."

6. Thomas A. LaVeist et al., "The Economic Burden of Racial, Ethnic, and Educational Health Inequities in the US," *JAMA* 329, no. 19 (May 2023): 1682–92, https://doi:10.1001/jama.2023.5965.

7. Paul Braff, "Moving from the National Negro Health Week to the National Public Health Week in the United States," *American Journal of Public Health* 110, no. 4 (April 2020): 470–74.

8. Paul Braff, "Moving from the National Negro Health Week."

9. Margaret M. Heckler, *Report of the Secretary's Task Force on Black and Minority Health*, Department of Health and Human Services (Washington, DC, 1985), https://www.minorityhealth.hhs.gov/assets/pdf/checked/1/ANDERSON .pdf. This report was coauthored by researcher Thomas E. Malone, who was the deputy director of the National Institutes of Health at the time this report was written.

Chapter 8. Treating Cancers, One Bill at a Time

1. Breast Cancer Program, H.B. 766, https://mgaleg.maryland.gov /mgawebsite/Search/Legislation?target=/1998rs/billfile/hb0766.htm.

2. Kathleen A. Mathias Chemotherapy Parity Act of 2012, H.B. 243, https:// mgaleg.maryland.gov/mgawebsite/Search/Legislation?target=/2012rs/billfile /hb0243.htm.

3. Margaret M. Heckler, *Report of the Secretary's Task Force on Black and Minority Health*, Department of Health and Human Services (Washington, DC, 1985), https://www.minorityhealth.hhs.gov/assets/pdf/checked/1/ANDERSON.pdf.

4. Oral Health Programs—Reducing Oral Cancer Mortality, H.B. 1184, https://mgaleg.maryland.gov/mgawebsite/Search/Legislation?target=/2000rs /billfile/hb1184.htm.

5. Heckler, *Report of the Secretary's Task Force on Black and Minority Health*.

6. Cigarette Restitution Fund Program, https://health.maryland.gov/phpa /crfp/pages/home.aspx.

7. Health Insurance—Mandated Benefits—Hospitalization and Home Visits Following a Mastectomy, H.B. 41, https://mgaleg.maryland.gov/mgawebsite /Search/Legislation?target=/2009rs/billfile/hb0041.htm.

Chapter 9. Health Care Disparities Prevention

1. Nursing Homes—Staffing, H.B. 784, https://mgaleg.maryland.gov /mgawebsite/Search/Legislation?target=/2000rs/billfile/hb0784.htm.

2. Margaret M. Heckler, *Report of the Secretary's Task Force on Black and Minority Health*, Department of Health and Human Services (Washington, DC, 1985), https://www.minorityhealth.hhs.gov/assets/pdf/checked/1/ANDERSON .pdf.

3. *Now Is the Time: An Action Agenda for Improving Black and Minority Health in Maryland: The Final Report of Maryland Governor's Commission on Black and Minority Health*, Maryland Department of Health and Mental Hygiene, Policy and Health Statistics Administration, Division of Policy Analysis (Baltimore, 1987), https://eric.ed.gov/?id=ED326585.

4. Brian D. Smedley, Adrienne Y. Stith, and Alan R. Nelson, *Unequal Treatment: Confronting Racial and Ethnic Disparities in Health Care* (Washington, DC: National Academies Press, 2003), https://pubmed.ncbi.nlm.nih.gov/2503 2386/.

5. Health Care Services Disparities Prevention Act, H.B. 883, https://mgaleg
.maryland.gov/mgawebsite/Search/Legislation?target=/2003rs/billfile/hb0883.htm.

6. Maryland Office of Minority Health and Health Disparities, H.B. 86,
https://mgaleg.maryland.gov/mgawebsite/Search/Legislation?target=/2004rs
/billfile/hb0086.htm.

7. Health Occupations—Cultural Competency Workgroup, H.B. 1295,
https://mgaleg.maryland.gov/mgawebsite/Search/Legislation?target=/2006rs
/billfile/hb1295.htm.

8. *National Stakeholder Strategy for Achieving Health Equity*, Office of
Minority Health, Maryland Department of Health, https://minorityhealth.hhs
.gov/npa/files/Plans/NSS/completenss.pdf.

Chapter 10. Affordable Health Insurance for All

1. "Effect of the Affordable Care Act in Maryland," Ballotpedia, https://
ballotpedia.org/Effect_of_the_Affordable_Care_Act_in_Maryland.

2. For the source of these statistics, see *ACA Implementation-Monitoring and
Tracking: Who Gained Health Insurance Coverage Under the ACA, and Where Do
They Live?* Robert Wood Johnson Foundation, December 2016, https://www
.urban.org/research/publication/who-gained-health-insurance-coverage-under
-aca-and-where-do-they-live. See also Thomas C. Buchmueller, Zachary M.
Levinson, Helen G. Levy, and Barbara L. Wolfe, "Effect of the Affordable Care
Act on Racial and Ethnic Disparities in Health Insurance Coverage," *American
Journal of Public Health* 106, no. 8 (2016 August): 1416–21, https://www.ncbi
.nlm.nih.gov/pmc/articles/PMC4940635/.

3. For the source of these statistics, see *ACA Implementation-Monitoring and
Tracking*.

See also Bowen Garrett and Anuj Gangopadhyaya, *Who Gained Health
Insurance Coverage under the ACA, and Where Do They Live?*, Urban Institute,
December 21, 2016, https://www.urban.org/research/publication/who-gained
-health-insurance-coverage-under-aca-and-where-do-they-live/view/full_report.

Chapter 11. How Government Policies Sometimes Fuel Disparities

1. "Viral Hepatitis," Centers for Disease Control and Prevention, https://
www.cdc.gov/hepatitis/index.htm.

2. Disease Prevention—Hepatitis A and B Education and Prevention
Program, H.B. 195, https://mgaleg.maryland.gov/mgawebsite/Search
/Legislation?target=/2003rs/billfile/hb0195.htm.

3. *Report of the State Advisory Council on Hepatitis C State of Maryland*,
January 2006, https://phpa.health.maryland.gov/OIDPCS/AVHPP/AVHPP%20
Documents/MACHCRptFnlE.pdf.

4. Maryland Medical Assistance Program and Health Insurance—
Coverage—Hepatitis C Drugs, S.B. 0943, https://mgaleg.maryland.gov
/mgawebsite/Legislation/Details/sb0943?ys=2018RS&search=True.

Chapter 12. Education Equity Is Health Equity

1. "Debunking Myths about Dyslexia," 2023, http://dyslexiahelp.umich.edu /parents/learn-about-dyslexia/what-is-dyslexia/debunking-common-myths -about-dyslexia.

2. Task Force to Study the Implementation of a Dyslexia Education Program, S.B. loo15, https://mgaleg.maryland.gov/mgawebsite/Legislation/Details /sb0015?ys=2015RS&search=True.

3. *Final Report of the Task Force to Study the Implementation of a Dyslexia Education Program*, December 31, 2016, https://msa.maryland.gov/megafile/msa /speccol/sc5300/sc5339/000113/021600/021654/20170046e.pdf.

4. Sonali Jhanjee, "Dyslexia and Substance Abuse: The Under-Recognized Link," *Indian Journal of Psychological Medicine* 37, no. 3 (July–September 2015): 374–75, https://doi.org/10.4103/0253-7176.162905.

5. *Report to Congress on the Prevention and Treatment of Co-occurring Substance Abuse Disorders and Mental Disorders: United States*, Substance Abuse and Mental Health Services Administration, 2002, https://archive.org/details /reporttocongressoooounse.

6. "Sickle Cell Disease: Causes and Risk Factors," NHLBI, NIH, August 30, 2023, https://www.nhlbi.nih.gov/health/sickle-cell-disease/causes.

7. *The Study of Adult Sickle Cell Disease in Maryland*, Department of Health and Mental Hygiene 2006 Legislative Report, https://phpa.health.maryland .gov/genetics/pdf/2006sicklecell_legis_rpt24.pdf.

8. *The Study of Adult Sickle Cell Disease in Maryland*.

9. *The Study of Adult Sickle Cell Disease in Maryland*.

10. *The Study of Adult Sickle Cell Disease in Maryland*.

11. Sickle Cell Disease—Statewide Steering Committee on Services for Adults with Sickle Cell Disease, H.B. 793, https://mgaleg.maryland.gov /mgawebsite/Search/Legislation?target=/2007RS/billfile/hb0793.htm.

Chapter 13. Maternal and Infant Mortality

1. Susan Scutti, "After Serena Williams Gave Birth, 'Everything Went Bad,'" January 11, 2018, http://CNN.com/2018/01/10/health/serena-williams-birth-c -section-olympia-bn/index.html.

2. Alice Park, "Beyonce Says She Had Toxemia during Her Pregnancy With Her Twins: Here's What That Means," *Time Magazine*, August 6, 2018, https:// time.com/5358684/beyonce-toxemia-preeclampsia/.

3. *Maryland Maternal Mortality Review Program 2018 Annual Report*, Maryland Department of Health, https://phpa.health.maryland.gov/documents/Health -General-Article-§13-1207-2018-Annual-Report-Maryland-Maternal-Mortality -Review.pdf.

4. "Preventing Pregnancy-Related Deaths," Centers for Disease Control and Prevention, April 26, 2023, https://www.cdc.gov/reproductivehealth/maternal -mortality/preventing-pregnancy-related-deaths.html.

5. Emily E. Petersen et al., "Racial/Ethnic Disparities in Pregnancy-Related Deaths—United States, 2007–2016," *MMWR* and *Morbidity and Mortality Weekly Report* 68 (2019): 762–65, https://www.cdc.gov/mmwr/volumes/68/wr/mm6835a3.htm.

6. *Study of Mortality Rates of African American Infants and Infants in Rural Areas: Report to the Senate Finance Committee and the House Health and Government Operations Committee*, Maryland Health Care Commission, November 2019, https://mhcc.maryland.gov/mhcc/pages/plr/plr/documents/IMRprtFINAL_10312019.pdf.

Chapter 14. Beyond Health Care

1. *Closing the Gap in a Generation: Health Equity through Action on the Social Determinants of Health—Final Report of the Commission on Social Determinants of Health*, World Health Organization, August 27, 2008, https://www.who.int/publications/i/item/WHO-IER-CSDH-08.1.

2. *Baltimore City 2017 Neighborhood Health Profile: Sandtown-Winchester/Harlem Park*, Baltimore City Health Department (Baltimore, MD, 2017), https://health.baltimorecity.gov/sites/default/files/NHP%202017%20-%2047%20Sandtown-Winchester-Harlem%20Park%20(rev%206-9-17).pdf.

3. "Maryland at a Glance, Economy, Unemployment, Unemployment Rates," Maryland Manual On-Line, August 24, 2023, https://msa.maryland.gov/msa/mdmanual/01glance/economy/html/unemployrates.html; "US Unemployment Rate 1991–2023," https://www.macrotrends.net/countries/USA/united-states/unemployment-rate#:~:text=U.S.%20unemployment%20rate%20for%202019,a%200.46%25%20decline%20from%202017.

4. Higher Education - Cyber Warrior Diversity Program - Revisions, S.B. 0432, https://mgaleg.maryland.gov/mgawebsite/Legislation/Details/sb0432?ys=2019RS&search=True.

5. *Workgroup on Health in All Policies, September 30, 2019 Report*, University of Maryland School of Public Health, Center for Health Equity, https://sph.umd.edu/sites/default/files/images/Sept%2030t%202019%20HiAP%20Report_Final%20(1).pdf.

Chapter 15. Lasting Legacy and Advocacy

1. Thomas A. LaVeist, Darrell Gaskin, and Patrick Richard, "Estimating the Economic Burden of Racial Health Inequalities in the United States," *International Journal of Health Services: Planning, Administration, Evaluation* 41, no. 2 (2011): 231–38, https://doi.org/10.2190/HS.41.2.c.

2. "Effects of the Coronavirus COVID-19 Pandemic (CPS)," Labor Force Statistics from the Current Population Survey, Bureau of Labor Statistics, November 2, 2022, https://.bls.gov/cps/effects-of-the-coronavirus-covid-19-pandemic.htm.

Black Psychiatrists of America, 60

Black women: breast cancer mortality rates, 94; first in Maryland House of Delegates, 32; first in US Congress, 32; first owner of a TV station, 52–53; maternal mortality rate, 152–57; racism toward, 29–30

Black Women Consciousness Raising Association, 51–52, 60

bladder cancer, 101

blockbusting, 38

blood transfusions, 131, 147–48

Bolt, Usain, 8

Bonnie (breast cancer patient), 103–6

Bon Secours Hospital, Baltimore, MD, 35–36, 46, 48, 69

Bootham Park Hospital School of Nursing, York, UK, 8, 16–18, 19–21, 28, 138

brain tumors, 101, 124–25

Branch, Harriet Bais, 93

Branch, Talmadge, 174

breast cancer diagnosis and treatment, 1–3, 93–98, 103–6, 117, 127–28

Bromwell, Thomas L., 108

Brown, Anna, 113–14

Brown, Michael, 162, 166

Brown, Roscoe C., 57–58

Brunson, Dorothy, 52–53

Burns, Emmett, 84

Burris, Henry, 110

CAIO. *See* Caribbean American Inter-Cultural Organization

Calomathi, Joseph, 12

Campbell, James "Jim," 51, 70, 71, 88

cancer, 62–63, 100–101, 101–2, 101–3, 111, 115–16, 117, 170–71. *See also specific types of cancer*

Cantler, James E., 121–22

Cardin, Ben, 120, 125, 185

cardiovascular disease, 62–63, 80, 99, 111, 112–14, 115–16, 155, 156, 164

CareFirst Inc., 58

Caribbean American Inter-Cultural Organization (CAIO), 43–44, 68, 69

Caribbean Heritage Month, 174

Carter, Jimmy, 58

Castile, Philando, 166

Castro, Fidel, 70

Center for Health Equity, 171

Centers for Disease Control and Prevention (CDC), 125, 154, 155, 156; National Breast and Cervical Cancer Early Detection Program, 94–95, 96; Pregnancy Mortality Surveillance System, 155

cervical cancer, 101, 117

Chappelle, Dave, 68

Chatman, Priscilla, 95, 97

chemotherapy, costs, 98–99

children: early childhood development, 161; health coverage under ACA, 127

Children of Sisyphus, The, 61

Chisholm, Shirley, 32, 56

chlorpyrifos, 170–71

Christensen, Donna, 54

Church Home and Hospital, Baltimore, MD, 35, 36

Cigarette Restitution Fund, 102–3, 115–16

cirrhosis, 62–63, 112, 131

civil rights movement, 23–24, 53, 60–70

Clarke, Yvette, 185

Clinton, Bill, 78, 95, 120

Clinton, Hillary, 122

Cockpit Country, Jamaica, 8–9, 12

College Board, College Level Examination Program (CLEP), 47

Collier, Maxie T., 52, 60

colon cancer, 101

colonoscopies, screening, 127–28

Commissioner of Baltimore City Department of Social Services, 82

Common Entrance Exam, 73

community activism, 43–46, 51–67

Community College of Baltimore County, 47

Community Health Resources Commission, 180–81

comprehensive care, 148

Congressional Black Caucus: Black Caucus Weekend, 174; Health Braintrust, 45, 54, 55–56

Congress on Health and Economic Disparities, 114

continuity of care, 26, 130, 150–51, 159

Coppin State University, 165, 184–85

Marshall, Thurgood, 185

Maryland Black Caucus Foundation: Black Caucus Weekend, 174; Senator of the Year Award, 174

Maryland Black Congress on Health, Law, and Economics, 59–60

Maryland Board of Public Works, 83

Maryland Dental Society, 59

Maryland Department of Health and Mental Hygiene, 58, 95, 132, 169, 171, 180–81; Electronic Reporting and Surveillance System (MERSS), 132–33; Family Health Administration, 117; *The Hospital Discharge Database of the Maryland Health Care Commission*, 148–49; Prevention and Health Promotion Administration, 103; Shirley Nathan-Pulliam Health Equity Lecture series, 184. *See also* Office of Minority Health and Health Disparities

Maryland Department of Housing, 172

Maryland Department of Human Resources, 169

Maryland Department of Public Safety and Correctional Services, 168–69

Maryland Department of Transportation, 172

Maryland General Assembly, 85; Appropriations Committee, 115–16; Environmental Matters Committee, 96; legislative districts, 84, 88; members of Caribbean descent, 173–74; Sickle Cell Day, 150. *See also* Maryland House of Delegates

Maryland Health Care Commission, *Study of Mortality Rates of African Americans Infants . . .* , 158–59

Maryland Health in All Policies Framework, 172

Maryland Health Services Cost Review Commission (HSCRC), 94–95

Maryland House of Delegates, 51, 59, 97, 182; Appropriations Committee, 88; Education, Health, and Environmental Affairs Committee, 108; Environmental Matters Committee, 96; first Black woman delegate, 32; Forty-Fourth District, 163–64, 173; Forty-Second District, 88; Health and Government Operations Committee, Minority Health Disparities Subcommittee, 124; Shirley Nathan-Pulliam's career in, 3, 32, 84–89; Social Services Commission, 88. *See also* legislative achievements, of Shirley Nathan-Pulliam

Maryland Medical Assistance Program, 135

Maryland Mental Health Coalition, Joint Workshop on Co-occurring Disorders, 146

Maryland Nurses Association, 44, 69

Maryland Port Administration, 86

Maryland Senate, 51, 88, 89, 95–96, 97, 107–8, 124, 182, 184; first Black woman member, 32; Shirley Nathan-Pulliam's career in, 32, 124, 137, 140–42, 170–71, 173–77

Maryland State Attorney, 51

Maryland State Department of Education, 142

Maryland State House, 85

Maryland State Medical Society, 134

Maryland Top 100 Woman award, 184

mastectomy, 2, 93, 104–6

maternal mortality, 152–57, 159

Maternal Mortality Review Program, 155–57

McCain, John, 123

McCready, Esther, 185

McDaniels, John P., 58

McDonald, Icy, 20

McDonald, LaQuan, 166

McKay, Claude, "The Negro's Tragedy," 136

McLeod, Millicent, 71

Medicaid, 82, 126, 127, 134, 135, 146, 148, 149, 169, 181

medical schools and education, 117–18, 119

Medicare, 148

MedStar Health, 58

Mental Health Association of Maryland, 146–47

mental health issues, 111, 159, 164; of Black men, 60–61; co-occurrence with substance abuse disorders, 145–47;